P9-AGI-975

J. LeBron McBride, PhD, MPH

Family Behavioral Issues in Health and Illness

"**T**his is an excellent resource to help health care professionals understand the powerful influences of their patients' family dynamics and how these factors can enhance or sabotage medical treatment. The work is written in a concise and well-organized manner.

This will be a helpful resource for graduate students in the health care fields to aid their understanding of clinical issues for families that range from life cycle issues and developmental markers to specific family systems concepts, such as boundaries, subsystems, scapegoating, and parentification. The work also identifies special family experiences such as divorce, bereavement, and substance abuse and the influence of these on the health and functioning of its members.

The author, through his selection of practical and focused content, creates a successful dialogue between the fields of family therapy and family medicine."

Craig A. Everett, PhD
Director, Arizona Institute
for Family Therapy;
Editor, *Journal of Divorce and Remarriage*;
Past President, American Association
for Marriage and Family Therapy

"**M**cBride's book is a comprehensive overview of families. A useful guide for family physicians as we frame the future of family medicine, we must also frame the future of families. Effective, quickly read, practical strategies for all family structures and problems. The sections on violence and divorce are particularly helpful. On any day, any family situation may arise; this would be a handy reference for anyone who works in the medical setting."

Peggy Wagner, PhD
Professor,
Department of Family Medicine,
Medical College of Georgia

More pre-publication
REVIEWS, COMMENTARIES, EVALUATIONS . . .

"**D**r. McBride's book provides a framework for the health care provider to address the family context of the patient's issue or problem. He does so by depicting the changing American family, presenting normal individual and family developmental stages, and describing the crises faced at different stages of development. Next he describes methods the health care provider can use to prevent difficulties in well-functioning individuals and families, and strategies for intervention or referral for families where dysfunction interferes with good patient care. He presents cases of common health care issues that involve family issues and incorporates tables and charts that suggest means of assessment and intervention regarding particular family issues such as parenting or dementia.

This book is essential reading for health care providers who want to build trust by communicating an understanding of the patient's health care challenges, and by marshalling resources to assist patients in keeping or getting well. This is a handy, easy-to-read guide, authored by a practitioner with years of experience working alongside health care providers of many types.

Of most value are sections describing typical issues encountered at each stage of the family life cycle, strains as-sociated with each stage, and suggestions for preventing difficulties at each stage. In addition, Dr. McBride describes the delicate challenge faced by the health care provider who wants to build patient-provider rapport while not taking sides or being drawn into family conflicts. He provides solutions that maintain trust while not alienating either side in a family conflict. Dr. McBride provides guidance for the most difficult of family issues such as violence, chronic or terminal illness, and substance abuse. Dr. McBride astutely depicts not only the difficulties encountered by traditional families but also by those families that vary from the traditional family structure such as blended and single-parent families, gay and lesbian families, adoptive families, families with infertility issues, and families who have immigrated from other countries. Health care providers are the obvious audience for this book, but others who may benefit are trainers of health care providers and health care center administrators seeking to improve care to patients and families."

Sylvia Shellenberger, PhD
Psychologist and Professor
of Family Medicine,
Mercer University School of Medicine

The Haworth Press
New York • London • Oxford

Family Behavioral Issues
in Health and Illness

HAWORTH Marriage and Family Therapy
Terry S. Trepper, PhD
Senior Editor

Psychotherapy with People in the Arts: Nurturing Creativity by Gerald Schoenewolf

Critical Incidents in Marital and Family Therapy: A Practitioner's Guide by David A. Baptiste Jr.

Clinical and Educational Interventions with Fathers edited by Jay Fagan and Alan J. Hawkins

Family Solutions for Substance Abuse: Clinical and Counseling Approaches by Eric E. McCollum and Terry S. Trepper

The Therapist's Notebook for Families: Solution-Oriented Exercises for Working with Parents, Children, and Adolescents by Bob Bertolino and Gary Schultheis

Between Fathers and Sons: Critical Incident Narratives in the Development of Men's Lives by Robert J. Pellegrini and Theodore R. Sarbin

Women's Stories of Divorce at Childbirth: When the Baby Rocks the Cradle by Hilary Hoge

Treating Marital Stress: Support-Based Approaches by Robert P. Rugel

An Introduction to Marriage and Family Therapy by Lorna L. Hecker and Joseph L. Wetchler

Solution-Focused Brief Therapy: Its Effective Use in Agency Settings by Teri Pichot and Yvonne M. Dolan

Becoming a Solution Detective: Identifying Your Client's Strengths in Practical Brief Therapy by John Sharry, Brendan Madden, and Melissa Darmody

Emotional Cutoff: Bowen Family Systems Theory Perspectives edited by Peter Titelman

Welcome Home! An International and Nontraditional Adoption Reader edited by Lita Linzer Schwartz and Florence W. Kaslow

Creativity in Psychotherapy: Reaching New Heights with Individuals, Couples, and Families by David K. Carson and Kent W. Becker

Understanding and Treating Schizophrenia: Contemporary Research, Theory, and Practice by Glenn D. Shean

Family Involvement in Treating Schizophrenia: Models, Essential Skills, and Process by James A. Marley

Transgender Emergence: Therapeutic Guidelines for Working with Gender-Variant People and Their Families by Arlene Istar Lev

Family Treatment of Personality Disorders: Advances in Clinical Practice edited by Malcolm M. MacFarlane

Unbecoming Mothers: The Social Production of Maternal Absence edited by Diana L. Gustafson

Therapy with Single Parents: A Social Constructionist Approach by Joan D. Atwood and Frank Genovese

Family Behavioral Issues in Health and Illness by J. LeBron McBride

When Adoptions Go Wrong: Psychological and Legal Issues of Adoption Disruption by Lita Linzer Schwartz

Family Behavioral Issues in Health and Illness

J. LeBron McBride, PhD, MPH

The Haworth Press
New York • London • Oxford

For more information on this book or to order, visit
http://www.haworthpress.com/store/product.asp?sku=5621

or call 1-800-HAWORTH (800-429-6784) in the United States and Canada
or (607) 722-5857 outside the United States and Canada

or contact orders@HaworthPress.com

Published by

The Haworth Press, Inc., 10 Alice Street, Binghamton, NY 13904-1580.

This book is an expanded version of a work that appeared as a monograph for the American Academy of Family Physicians, used by permission: McBride JL. *Family Behavioral Issues.* Monograph Edition No. 285, AAFP Home Study. Leawood, KS: American Academy of Family Physicians, February 2003.

PUBLISHER'S NOTES
The development, preparation, and publication of this work has been undertaken with great care. However, the Publisher, employees, editors, and agents of The Haworth Press are not responsible for any errors contained herein or for consequences that may ensue from use of materials or information contained in this work. The Haworth Press is committed to the dissemination of ideas and information according to the highest standards of intellectual freedom and the free exchange of ideas. Statements made and opinions expressed in this publication do not necessarily reflect the views of the Publisher, Directors, management, or staff of The Haworth Press, Inc., or an endorsement by them.

Identities and circumstances of individuals discussed in this book have been changed to protect confidentiality.

Cover design by Lora Wiggins.

Library of Congress Cataloging-in-Publication Data

McBride, J. LeBron.
    Family behavioral issues in health and illness / J. LeBron McBride.
      p. ; cm.
    Rev. ed. of: Family behavioral issues. 2003.
    Includes bibliographical references and index.
    ISBN-13: 978-0-7890-2943-0 (hc. : alk. paper)
    ISBN-10: 0-7890-2943-X (hc. : alk. paper)
    ISBN-13: 978-0-7890-2944-7 (pbk. : alk. paper)
    ISBN-10: 0-7890-2944-8 (pbk. : alk. paper)
    1. Family—Health and hygiene—United States. 2. Family—United States—Psychological aspects. 3. Family medicine—United States. 4. Life cycle, Human—Health aspects. I. McBride, J. LeBron. Family behavioral issues. II. Title.
    [DNLM: 1. Family—psychology—United States. 2. Family Health —United States. 3. Socioeconomic Factors—United States.
WS 105.5.F2 M478f 2006]
RA418.5.F3M42 2006
613—dc22

                                          2005024738

CONTENTS

Foreword

If you are picking up this book and debating whether you should read it or purchase it, we would like you to figure out a way to prop the book open to this page, put your hands under your legs, and sit quietly. Now, take a minute to map out the back of your hands in your mind's eye. Where are the moles, the freckles, and the scars? Trace the pattern of veins as they web their way across your hand. Picture the wrinkles around each knuckle. What are their shapes and patterns?

When you have done this, pull out the backs of your hands and tell us how well you really knew them. Were certain scars a different size or location than you remembered? Were the veins and freckles the color and depth you remembered? Were your wrinkles in the configurations you pictured them, or perhaps wanted them?

Understanding our families is similar to knowing the back of our hands. We think we know them better than we actually do. Each of us is raised in a family that is the foundation and centerpiece of our existence for the first couple of decades of life. We then pursue development of another family—either formally through marriage or informally through choice. In these families we experience great joy and profound crises. We feel incredible intimacy and are overwhelmed with the enormous pain of separation. As we travel across the ridges and through the crannies of life we start to feel as though we know our families—in fact, we know our families well—at least at some level.

But like the backs of our hands, we may not know the scars and wrinkles of family as well as we could or perhaps even should. Each family has its own unique set of patterns and systems. Ac-

Family Behavioral Issues in Health and Illness
Published by The Haworth Press, Inc., 2006. All rights reserved.
doi:10.1300/5621_a

quiring the ability to fully assess these and completely understand them is not possible. For those working in health care, a solid base of knowledge, skills, and attitudes concerning family is required. As this book so clearly reminds us, family relationships have a profound impact on health and illness. The more deeply we understand them the better we can guide those with whom we work toward a more complete well-being.

Family Behavioral Issues in Health and Illness is an excellent foundational reference detailing the connections between family and health. It should be required reading for all those who deal with patients from a holistic or complete health perspective. We have read many books on behavioral epidemiology and the relationship of the social environment to health, and have yet to see a more useable work in this area. For a short text, Dr. McBride does a superb job of providing a concise and surprisingly complete summary of family systems theory, basic family assessment, and the typical family life cycle. He then reminds us of the variations that occur in families and the specific health care issues that may arise in each circumstance. Finally, with great skill he reviews a series of particular difficulties that families may experience and the connections each of these may have on health and illness.

In the narrative as well as through exhibits and figures, the reader is provided with an inclusive list of the most important aspects of family to consider when providing care. The use of case studies brings a practical real life quality that draws us in. The book is heavily referenced throughout, providing the scientist with confidence in its message, and the student with further resources should a particular area need to be studied in greater depth. Every health care provider should consider purchasing this text as a regular reference when issues of family interact with health and illness— and they do all the time.

As health care professional educators in medicine, nursing, and public health as well as a family who has experienced the pain of separation and the difficulties of a child with a major disability, we were delighted to read this book and recognize its contribution to the literature on family and health. We heartily recommend it to educators, learners, parents, and family members. We look forward to being able to provide it to our students and are already using it to remind ourselves of the realities of the backs of our hands—complete with scars, wrinkles, and so much more to discover.

Wayne S. Dysinger, MD, MPH, FAAFP
Chair, Department of Preventive Medicine
School of Medicine

June N. Dysinger, MN, MPH, RN, CNM
Course Coordinator, Health Promotion Across the Lifespan
School of Nursing
Loma Linda University

ABOUT THE AUTHOR

J. LeBron McBride, PhD, MPH, is Director of Behavioral Medicine and Clerkship Director, as well as a faculty member at Floyd Medical Center's Family Medicine Residency Program in Rome, Georgia. He is an Associate Clinical Professor at Mercer University School of Medicine in Macon, Georgia, Assistant Clinical Professor at the Medical College of Georgia in Augusta, and senior minister of the First Christian Church (Disciples of Christ) in Rome, Georgia. Dr. McBride is the author of *Spiritual Crisis: Surviving Trauma to the Soul* (Haworth), *Living Faithfully with Disappointment in the Church* (Haworth), and the forthcoming *Pastoral Care from the Pulpit: Meditations of Hope and Encouragement* (Haworth).

Preface

This book is a basic introduction to family issues that are important in health care. Although more extensive works are available, this book meets the need for a concise introduction and one that can be a supplemental text in the training of persons with various health orientations and disciplines. Within the interior of families may be found the greatest promoters for health and happiness or, on the other hand, the cruelest and most violently destructive environments known to humankind. This work will assist readers in better understanding the dynamics of the powerful institution we call the family and its impact upon health and illness. Ignoring the influence of the family can result in less than optimal medical treatment while incorporating its influence can greatly enhance treatment.

Therefore, it is vital for health care professionals to consider the family in which a patient resides. In at least one branch of health care, family medicine, the family has been viewed as the context for medical care. Although the emphasis on the family has not always been implemented fully, even in family medicine (Kahn, 2004; McBride, 2004) an understanding of the family's impact upon health and illness should be integrated as an important concept of any primary care model. Historically, an emphasis on the family context of care may include the following beliefs:

1. The family is the primary social context for health care.
2. Patients' individual problems are family problems.
3. The patient's family is potentially the health care provider's greatest ally.
4. The health care provider's own family life is a component of patient encounters.
5. Family-oriented primary care treatment can be an effective way to help patients and families.

Family Behavioral Issues in Health and Illness
Published by The Haworth Press, Inc., 2006. All rights reserved.
doi:10.1300/5621_b

6. Family-oriented medical care requires education beyond the normal training of health care providers. (Doherty and Baird, 1983, pp. 3-6)

Such tenets can be very practical and can improve patient care. Families continue to be the primary environment in which most patients develop and are introduced to beliefs about culture, religion, health and illness, and overall attitudes about living (Butler and Lang, 2001). A large body of evidence reveals the effectiveness of family interventions in health care and strongly supports a family-systems approach to medicine (Campbell, 2001). Medical professionals can better accomplish interventions, even in a busy practice, as they become more adept and knowledgeable about family dynamics and the critical pivotal points of family life. Knowledge of where a patient is in the family life cycle as well as assessing and anticipating family dynamics may be the key to successful treatment. Family-oriented care may prove to provide the most comprehensive patient care as well as the most effective management of time and resources. Dr. Macaran Baird, a respected authority in the field of family medicine, stated, "Attending to the psychosocial dimensions and family dimensions of health care reduces costs as well as improves clinical aspects of care" (Baird, 2001, p. 61). This book addresses family behavioral issues that can assist the health care worker with patient care from a family-oriented context.

Acknowledgments

I am indebted to those medical students, family medicine residents, and faculty physicians with whom I have worked for more than a decade. You have assisted me in understanding the complexity of medical care within the constraints of our modern medical system. Many of you do exceptional and sensitive work incorporating an understanding of the family context even with time pressures always nipping at your heels. You and other such health care providers are unrecognized heroes.

I also recognize what patients have taught me about the illness experience. I have witnessed the agony of those with diseased and broken bodies and wounded souls. Many times I have been amazed by the fortitude and tenacity of the human spirit. Often the resilience of those patients confronted by overwhelming pain and suffering and the tender support of them by their families is spectacular. Such patients and their families also are my heroes.

The original version of this work appeared as a monograph for the American Academy of Family Physicians and I am indebted to those who assisted with it in the original format. Jo Ann Rosenfeld, MD, served as the associate medical editor for the monograph and Cindy Moreland did a wonderful job as senior editor.

I gratefully appreciated having two medical professionals who do family health care, Wayne Dysinger, MD, and June Dysinger, MN, write the foreword for this book. It was wonderful having a couple who share the joys and trials of family life together and who incorporate the family context into their work, introduce *Family Behavioral Issues in Health and Illness*. Appreciation also

Family Behavioral Issues in Health and Illness
Published by The Haworth Press, Inc., 2006. All rights reserved.
doi:10.1300/5621_c

goes to The Haworth Press and Dawn Krisko for her copyediting work.

Without the assistance of those acknowledged here, this work would not have reached its final destination. However, the responsibility for any shortcoming of the final product falls fully upon me.

Chapter 1

The Changing American Family

DEFINITION

The U.S. Census Bureau defines a family household as two or more individuals living together and related by blood, marriage, or adoption. However, family scholars make this definition more comprehensive by including individuals who choose an arrangement for living together that involves some type of emotional or economic support. For example, leading family researchers David Olson and John DeFrain (2000) describe family as, "two or more people who are committed to each other and who share intimacy, resources, decision-making responsibilities, and values" (p. 10). Although family is defined differently by various groups and individuals, in all families—even considering the current diversity of family life—repeating patterns of interactions and repeating influences are evident among family members. These interactions influence the health of each family member. The family system is an important—possibly the most important—context in which to view health care and behavior.

Most medical professionals realize that the North American family is evolving, but the magnitude of change in recent decades may not be realized. Some of these changes and statistics include the following (Campbell and McDaniel, 2001; Fields, 2001; Hobbs and Stoops, 2002; Whitehead and Popenoe, 2005):

1. The number of individuals who are unmarried and cohabiting has increased rapidly; cohabitation now precedes more than

Family Behavioral Issues in Health and Illness
Published by The Haworth Press, Inc., 2006. All rights reserved.
doi:10.1300/5621_01

half of all first marriages. Among young people, in particular, acceptance of cohabitation has significantly increased.

2. The number of marriages in America is declining. The percentage of the population over fifteen that is married has decreased 14 percentage points since 1960. However, currently 85 to 90 percent of the population marries at least once. Being married has repeatedly been shown to be a possitive variable in health.

3. Individuals are marrying at a later age. In 1970, the median age at first marriage was twenty years for women and twenty-three years for men. Currently, the ages for first marriage are twenty-five years for women and twenty-seven years for men; these are oldest ages for first marriage in our history.

4. The divorce rate, after increasing rapidly from the 1960s and reaching a peak in the 1980s, has decreased to approximately 50 percent.

5. The traditional model of the father working outside the home and the mother staying home with children occurs only in approximately 25 percent of families.

6. The percentage of children living in two-parent households has declined. In recent years 69 percent of American children lived with two parents, down from 88 percent in 1988.

7. The number of single-parent families was only 9 percent in 1960 but has now climbed to around 28 percent. The increase in single-parent families is one of the most significant trends that affects children.

8. Recently, 34.6 percent of all births were to unmarried women; in 1960 the percentage of all births to unmarried women was 5.3 percent.

9. The percentage of children living apart from their biological fathers has more than doubled since 1960, from 17 percent to an estimated 34 percent.

10. The poverty rate for children dropped recently to 16 percent, its lowest point in twenty years. The poverty rate increased in 2003 and 2004 to 17.8 percent.

11. Senior citizens (adults age sixty-five years and older) made up 8 percent of the population in 1950. By 2020, this group will constitute 17 percent of the population. In the most re-

cent decade the senior citizens group increased more than tenfold.

12. In the most recent census, approximately 600,000 households were identified as same-sex, unmarried partner households. (Because of the different variables and processes used, it is not possible to compare this accurately with previous census reports.)

13. The number of Hispanic children in the United States has increased faster than any other racial or ethnic group, from 9 percent of the population in 1980 to approximately 16 percent currently. By 2020, projections are that 1 in 5 children in the United States will be of Hispanic origin. The Hispanic population has more than doubled in size since 1990.

These statistics are important because they indicate potential changes in family structure, support structures, and possible stressors patients may be experiencing. Health care providers would do well to incorporate knowledge of major family life changes into their patient care.

The nuclear family, as it has existed in Western culture since the industrial revolution, is not the historically predominant form of the family. Typically, in many cultures, the family has been less isolated and more community-based. Health care providers must realize that the family model or structure they have been raised within may not fit with many actual practices of family life. To be most responsive and effective with diverse patient populations, providers must understand the patient's family context, which may be quite different from their own.

FAMILY SYSTEMS THEORY

The dominant model in medicine for assessing families is family systems theory. This approach incorporates interactions, relationships, and feedback loops. Rather than a linear causality, such as A causes B causes C, family systems theory incorporates the effects of B and C on A and various interactions and feedback loops (Figure 1.1). The linear, cause and effect, approach predisposes a

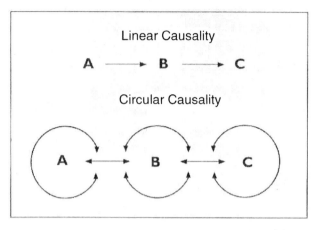

FIGURE 1.1. Linear versus circular causality.

closed system where relationships are fixed and not changing; systems model predisposes an open system, similar to a family, where relationships are in flux and continually influencing each other (Zubialde and Aspy, 2001).

The family systems approach is also referred to as circular causality. Much medical training has focused on cause and effect, often reducing physical disease to the central "cause." This has produced differential diagnoses, but it is less effective when used with family and psychosocial dynamics and influences. For a holistic approach to health care, consider health and illness being influenced in the wider "interactional field," such as the family, rather than in individual isolation (Christie-Seely, 1984).

George's visit to your office shortly after his fortieth birthday is prompted by his wife. He is feeling well, and his only concern is the weight he has put on during the last few years. You make note of his high blood pressure, obesity, and family history of diabetes, and decide to screen him for diabetes. The screen reveals that George has type 2 diabetes. You discuss ways to modify his diet, the importance of exercise, and the relationship of obesity to diabetes with George. George follows up with his regularly scheduled appointments for the next two years but makes no progress with lifestyle modifications. Finally, you recommend that he bring his wife with him to the next office visit. With his wife present, you give the same advice about the dangers of uncontrolled diabetes and the importance of lifestyle modifications. Six months later, George's wife accompanies him to your office, without your invitation, and reports that she has been shopping for the proper foods and that she and George have begun a walking program. George has lost twenty pounds, and his blood pressure levels are improved.

Family systems theory is based on the premise that individuals should be viewed in the context of interactions, transitions, and relationships inherent in the family rather than in isolation. This is similar to acknowledging that any organ of the body is interrelated and interactive with other organ systems and must be assessed in this wider context. What affects one person affects the entire system, and what affects the family system affects each member. "The whole is greater than the sum of the parts" is an often-quoted statement in family systems theory. One cannot look at each member of the family individually and understand the family. We must include the interactions and relationships of the family as a whole to understand it. Most medical office visits are with individual patients, but appreciating each patient's family context and influence enables providers to give more comprehensive and effective care.

Too often, health care providers ignore the effect of family dynamics on wellness and sickness. The illness experience is multifactorial, and the family context is a major context for care. Some of the many factors that impact health are shown in Figure 1.2. Instead of counseling a patient with diabetes about dietary changes without talking to other family members, it is better to include other individual family members, especially the one who does the grocery shopping or cooking.

THE FAMILY AND ITS INFLUENCE ON HEALTH

Families function in various ways to influence health. Although not completely understood, family relationships can greatly affect areas of health, such as physical and psychologic well-being, recovery from physical and mental illness, compliance, and longevity (Doherty and Baird, 1983; Campbell and McDaniel, 2001; Weihs et al., 2002). Major pathways by which family and social relationships

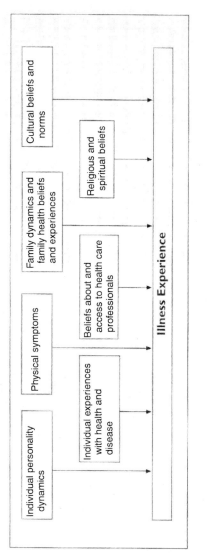

FIGURE 1.2. Contributions to the illness experience. *Source:* Adapted from McBride. 1998;109.

6

can influence health are through direct biologic pathways (e.g., infectious diseases, toxic environments, and shared genes); behavior pathways (i.e., lifestyle behaviors); and psychophysiologic pathways (e.g., cognition and emotions resulting in physiologic responses) (Campbell and McDaniel, 2001). Specific examples of the correlation between family and health include the following:

1. Families tend to share the same lifestyle protective or risk behaviors in areas such as diet, exercise, conflict, stress reactions, and support.
2. Of all types of support provided by families, emotional support (e.g., empathy, a listening ear, a sense of belonging, and a sense that one is cared about) has the most influence on health outcomes.
3. Being married or being in a relationship has been shown to have a protective factor on health.
4. Consistent links have been established between disease management and family processes, such as family closeness and connectedness, caregiver coping skills, and clear family organization.
5. Children with household family members who smoke have higher rates of upper respiratory infections, ear infections, and asthma, and adults with household members who smoke have higher rates of lung cancer.
6. Specific genetic diseases, such as hemophilia and Huntington's disease, and inherited risk for coronary artery disease, asthma, and cancer are correlated with family influences. (Campbell and McDaniel, 2001, pp. 16-19)

In the course of providing (or even when disregarding) emotional, spiritual, relational, and physical care, families can have a strong influence on the habits, beliefs, attitudes, behaviors, and knowledge of patients. Therefore, the family provides one of the best resources for disease prevention, intervention, and treatment. In many instances, to ignore the context of the family is to provide less than optimal medical care. Assessing a patient's family dynamics and influences can offer essential clues to understanding and developing strategies for intervening in a holistic approach to health care.

BASIC FAMILY ASSESSMENT

Families are complex, but knowledge of a few concepts about families can provide a basic understanding of their functioning. Just as medical systems have characteristics that assist with understanding, so do families. Basic family assessment tools found in family therapy literature include descriptions of boundaries, roles, rules, subsystems, triangles, scapegoating, parentification, disengagement and enmeshment, and communication (Everett, 2000). These dynamics are familiar to most individuals at some level of consciousness. However, by defining them, a more conscious awareness can occur so that they become a resource for assessment and intervention.

Boundaries

The Robins' represent a family with diffuse boundaries. Their household is similar to Grand Central Station with people coming and going constantly. Friends and relatives drop in whenever they are having financial difficulties, and then leave after staying a few weeks. The main household members comprise the mother, Jennifer, and her three children from three previous relationships. Jennifer ran away from her family of origin at a young age, so she is always kind to individuals in need of shelter. Various adults have kept the younger children while Jennifer works, but there has been no consistency in caregivers. The eldest child, now age seventeen, stays away for days or weeks at a time, then brings one of her friends into the home for a temporary stay. Sometimes, Jennifer takes the children to a friend's house at the last moment for child care. Her twelve-year-old daughter, Sara, is taken to the family practice clinic because of continued enuresis. A urine culture reveals a sexually transmitted disease, and child protective services becomes involved. It is discovered that one of the many visitors in the home had sexually abused Sara while being in charge of child care.

Boundaries are similar to invisible lines that reveal where separations occur. Boundaries determine the family's give-and-take with the external environment. They also indicate who is in the family and who is not. Very diffuse family boundaries that allow individuals to constantly come and go can be problematic, making it difficult to know who is a member of the family and who is not.

Diffuse boundaries may give little protection and stability to children and can cause the family to become extremely chaotic and vulnerable. *Closed boundaries* can isolate the family and allow for little outside assistance and influence.

Families in which there is domestic abuse and violence often have closed boundaries. Closed boundaries may severely limit family members' ability to seek medical care, except in emergencies. A healthy family needs to have boundaries that are flexible enough to allow movement back and forth according to the needs of the family system. For example, many couples initially have relatively closed boundaries when they are establishing their relationship. This usually gives way to more open boundaries as they progress in their relationship. In some families, the family health care provider is regarded as almost a member of the family, while in others the health care provider is kept firmly at a distance from any knowledge about the family.

Roles

Roles describe the functions and tasks that family members perform in the system. Often, roles can be well defined, such as when one member is clearly the "health expert" and caregiver in the family. This person may determine how and when family members receive health care. The health care provider must seek an alliance with the health expert of the family, or suggestions made by the health care provider may be sabotaged. Traditional gender roles fluctuate in our society, and these changes may create conflict and misunderstanding.

Rules

Rules define the behaviors of family members. All families have rules, although many may be unspoken. Rules may determine when a person goes to a health care provider. Some families have a rule that you see a health care provider only if you are "on your deathbed," while others have a rule that you see a health care provider for any ache or pain.

Subsystems

Subsystems, such as the spousal, parental, sibling, and parent-child subsystems, are components of family structures. At times, the family health care provider must bring in other members of a family subsystem. An example of when this might be appropriate is incorporating another child in the sibling subsystem into an office visit to assist the health care provider in understanding a child with depression. Family scholars generally consider a functional spousal subsystem in a two-parent family to be critical to the balance of the family system. The previous descriptors of family are referred to as family structure elements since they are the organizational pieces of the family and what we witness as we observe the family. The following descriptors are referred to as family process elements since they are interactional issues in family life (Nichols and Everett, 1986).

Triangulation

Triangulation refers to the way that a third individual often is pulled into an interaction when tension exists between two individuals. Triangulation helps lessen the tension between the two individuals. A classic example is when a child becomes the scapegoat for tension in the parental relationship. By focusing on the child, the parents find an issue—the child's behavior—on which they can be united. (Scapegoating and parentification can be examples of triangulation in some cases.)

Scapegoating

Scapegoating is a process where tension or conflict in the family is assigned to one family member. The family scapegoat may be a member who acts out the tension in a setting outside the family and who becomes a unifying focus for other family members. Individuals who are made scapegoats can be given the role of "troublemaker" or "rebellious teen" and may be brought to the family health care provider for assessment.

Parentification

Parentification occurs when a child is pulled into a parental subsystem or given a parental role. It also can occur when one spouse parents the other. In a family system where there is a particular need for younger children to be cared for by an older child, parentification also can occur. Another example is when a parent does not keep a boundary between the child and parental subsystems and makes the child a confidant about adult matters or for needy emotional comfort. Parentification also may occur when a parent is physically or emotionally impaired and the child has to take responsibility for the household or the disabled parent. Health care providers should note such dynamics and help ensure that the child maintains proper peer relationships and appropriate developmental-level activities. Children who have been extremely parentified can be subject to depression, alienation, and isolation from other siblings and peers.

Disengagement and Enmeshment

Disengagement and enmeshment describe the boundaries between individuals in the family. *Disengagement* refers to boundaries between family members that are stronger than usual. Family members may not be aware of what is going on with each other and may not provide much support to each other.

Conversely, *enmeshment* describes the existence of few or loose boundaries between family members. In extreme cases, it refers to a lack of boundaries between family members. This can lead to "everybody knowing each other's business" and emotional states being shared throughout the family. Enmeshed families are more supportive of each other. However, in extreme cases, autonomy and individuality in these families are restricted. Although disengagement and enmeshment can vary according to culture, the extremes present greater dysfunction. Health care providers should be observant about these dynamics in families, which will enable them to anticipate support or lack of support for sick members and potential problems with family members soliciting assistance when necessary.

Communication Style

Communication is often a major point of misunderstanding and conflict in relationships. The family health care provider will notice patterns in how family members communicate. What tone do they use with each other? Do they appear to really hear each other? Who is the family spokesperson? Who speaks for whom? Is there congruence between the content of what is being said, the context of what is being said, and the way it is being said? Communication is not just verbal; it is largely nonverbal. Patients' body language can reveal much, especially when they are interacting with other family members. An example of this would be when domestic violence is present in a relationship. A husband, simply with eye contact, can communicate to his wife that he expects her to be silent while he speaks for her.

The aforementioned family assessment concepts can be invaluable in helping health care providers determine how to approach family members, communicate with them, and serve their health needs. Health care providers can adjust their approach and intervene when necessary based on family dynamics and better determine what anticipatory guidance may be necessary.

Additional important and influential factors in family life include the following:

- History of emotional trauma and loss
- Religious and spiritual heritage and family participation
- Cultural, racial, and ethnic background
- Health and illness experiences and beliefs
- Financial and economic resources
- Community involvement
- Substance abuse history
- Overall life beliefs

THE FAMILY GENOGRAM

Another useful tool for assessing and monitoring family functioning and family health is the genogram, which is a type of family tree made by using symbols. Three uses of the genogram in family practice are systemic record keeping, rapport building, and providing medical management and preventive health (McGold-rick et al., 1999). Genograms can help health care providers iden-tify complex patterns in families and provide a quick reminder of family dynamics, health issues, and concerns. In a review of litera-ture on genograms, Linda Papadopoulos and Robert Bor state that "genograms provide physicians with a diagnostic tool, which takes into account the possible causes and effects of illness. . . . Further research is needed to establish the usefulness and efficacy of genograms in counselling and medical practice" (Papadopoulos et al., 1997, p. 26).

A basic genogram can be completed gradually during a few ses-sions. A separate section at the back or front of every established patient's chart might include a genogram that can be updated as significant events occur. A genogram also can serve as a reminder for timing of anticipatory guidance regarding upcoming, critical family life cycle transition points. Basic symbols used in geno-grams and a sample genogram are given in Figure 1.3.

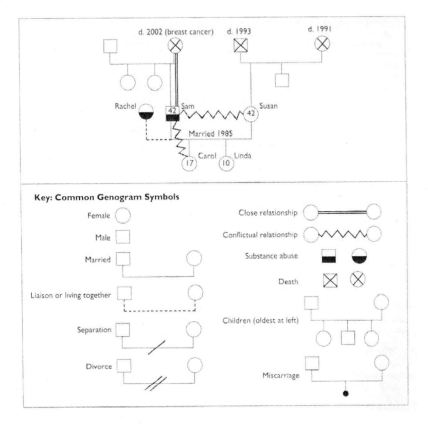

FIGURE 1.3. The genogram. *Note:* Sam and Susan have been married for eighteen years. They have a seventeen-year-old daughter, Carol, who is brought to the family physician's office because of difficulty sleeping, loss of interest in her usual activities, and sadness. Another daughter is age ten and is apparently doing fine. The paternal grandmother died one year ago of breast cancer (Sam was very close to his mother), and the maternal grandparents have been deceased several years. Both Susan and Carol speak of their conflict with Sam and complain of his lack of involvement in the family. Sam has had an affair recently, and both Sam and Rachel (the woman with whom he had the affair) have problems with substance abuse.

Chapter 2

The Family Life Cycle

As you complete your last weeks of practice before retirement, you find yourself reflecting upon your history with many of your patients. Today, Anita came in for her last visit with you. She first saw you when you were a resident. In fact, you delivered her first two children when you were in the residency program. You remember the joy Anita experienced at the births and the satisfaction you felt about the deliveries as a young resident. After you graduated, she became a patient in your practice and has remained with the practice for thirty-five years. You have even cared for her young grandchildren. Anita has experienced personal tragedy over the years. One of her children was killed in a car accident. You had young children at the time and remember how intensely the tragedy affected you. You provided brief supportive counseling as a component of Anita's office visits for several years after that.

Anita's husband left her just as her eldest child was entering adolescence. She was barely able to hang on and her daughter entered a troubled adolescence. She developed several physical problems and was treated for depression during that period, but she somehow persevered and eventually remarried. Anita has held several rather difficult jobs, but she has endured them all with little complaint. Now she is enjoying being a grandparent and appears to be in a good place in her life. You reflect on Anita's overall resilience and feel that you somehow played a small part in assisting her during the pivotal points in her life journey.

One way of understanding families is by examining the transitions the family experiences—the family life cycle. Usually, stages of the life cycle are based on family members entering and exiting because of marriage or cohabitation, death, a child being added to the family, or a young adult leaving the parental home. Although some life cycle events are fairly predictable based on age and sociocultural influences, recognizing the great diversity in lifestyles, family formations, and behaviors that exist today is important.

Family Behavioral Issues in Health and Illness
Published by The Haworth Press, Inc., 2006. All rights reserved.
doi:10.1300/5621_02

Variations in the life cycle experience also occur among ethnic groups, genders, divorced families, adoptive families, and families of different educational and economic levels. One stereotype should not be viewed as normal nor should all variations be viewed as abnormal.

The family life cycle consists of the following six stages:

1. Single young adulthood
2. Joining (the new couple)
3. The family with young children
4. The family with adolescents (which may also include providing care for the older generation)
5. The family launching children and moving on
6. The family in later life (Carter and McGoldrick, 1999, p. 2)

This orderly progression of stages is not always so well defined in reality, but it provides a good framework from which to think about life transitions. Finally, health care providers must not assume pathology if a family's life cycle does not fit this particular framework. All family members may not experience each stage, and the timing of some stages may vary more today than in past generations.

The life cycle stages are critical transition points and points of change and adaptation. When a family system is inflexible and cannot maintain balance between stability and change, it may become dysfunctional. For example, the rules and roles in a family when a child is age three must be quite different from when that child is age sixteen. Otherwise, the family can be like a horse and buggy attempting to travel down an interstate.

Life cycle transitions may stress the family system. Life cycle stages may intersect other patient issues. Health care providers may use anticipatory guidance to assist patients in navigating life-cycle transitions and adjustments. Patients who anticipate probable changes and stressors have an added resource at their disposal.

THE SINGLE YOUNG ADULT

Many young adults reach independence and decide to move out of the parental household. This life transition usually involves compromise and negotiation with their family of origin. In some families, this physical and emotional separation is so difficult that the young person or another family member will have a physical or emotional crisis. This crisis may keep the family unit in the same household for a longer period of time, especially if the young adult plays a critical role in maintaining the parents' marriage.

Another significant stressor is developing a career. Obtaining proper training or education may keep the young adult financially dependent on the parents. Deciding which career path to take can be an area of conflict between parents and children. In some families, there is tremendous pressure to pursue a certain career, such as parents wanting their children to follow career paths they wish they had taken. Family expectations may exist, such as expecting the eldest male in the family to follow the father's career or take over the family business. Other young adults may have no guidance from their parents and may look to accessible professionals, such as their health care provider, for some counsel in this area.

Setting up a household may be difficult for some young adults. They may have unrealistic desires and begin to live beyond their means. Decisions regarding boundaries and intimacy become paramount during this stage. The young adult has to decide how involved he or she wants to become with dating partners and whether or not this may involve living together or marriage. Rearrangement of the family cycle also may occur when the young adult returns to the parents' home because of divorce, difficulty maintaining a household, loss of job or income, or illness.

Lack of health insurance may be a major health concern when young adults are no longer covered by the parents' insurance policy and do not yet have coverage at their own workplace. Other health concerns are sexually transmitted diseases and contraception. With the threat of sexually transmitted diseases, especially acquired immunodeficiency syndrome (AIDS), young adults may need additional information on protected sexual practices. In addition, education about injury prevention, particularly motor vehicle accidents, is important in this age group.

THE NEW COUPLE

Although the age at first marriage is rising, cohabitation is becoming more prevalent in the United States and in the Western world. Most individuals still marry at some point in early adulthood. Individuals who marry as teenagers are much more likely to divorce. Some young adults use marriage to separate themselves emotionally from their parents, which may indicate that they have entered into the marriage to obtain emotional distance from their family of origin. As a result, these individuals may put too much pressure on their marital partners because of the neediness projected to that partner.

In American society, coupling and marriage have become endowed with many idealizations that place tremendous pressure on couple relationships. Therapists use the term *romantic idealization* to describe the illusions that come with the initial tendency to be blinded to a partner's faults. Although some religious institutions promote or require premarital counseling for individuals who plan to marry, many couples are not interested in counseling at this stage and often do not seek it. Health care providers can be instrumental in encouraging couples to seek counseling so that they have an opportunity to discuss major areas of couple life with a neutral third party. Romantic idealization can be a positive component of coupling and bonding if it is not extreme. However, when there is an extreme need by either partner for the other one to compensate for major deficits in his or her own personality, problems are likely to occur. Normally, romantic idealization becomes more realistic within a year or two after coupling. In individuals with personality disorders, such as borderline personality disorder, the romantic idealization can disappear quickly and dramatically and the partner may then be perceived in a totally negative manner.

As the romantic idealization evolves and becomes more balanced, the couple has to deal with increasingly realistic differences and make adjustments. Balancing individual needs and those of the marital relationship is an area of potential misunderstanding and conflict, especially for new couples. Health care providers can assist with normalizing relationships by asking appropriate questions like, "How is your family life going?" This can give patients opportunities to share confidential feelings. Young adults may benefit from hearing that relationships take work and adjustment and that healthy negotiation and conflict are part of good relationships.

Fertility, sexuality, and contraception are other issues for young adult couples. Many couples are having children at a later age than previous generations. Approximately 20 percent of women are older than age thirty when they give birth to their first child compared to 7 percent in 1960 (Johnson and Downs, 2005). The options for contraception, fertility, parenting, and adoption are varied today, and health care providers can educate and encourage the couple to make a decision that is reasonable for them.

THE FAMILY WITH YOUNG CHILDREN

The entry of a child into a family often is a dramatic transition for a couple. The anticipation of and buildup to the birth can be the focus of the couple's life during the entire pregnancy. Unfortunately, when domestic abuse is involved, the violence does not stop when the woman is pregnant, and in some cases, the abuse escalates (Hamberger, 2001). An appropriate question to ask during prenatal visits may be, "Sometimes, even with the joys of pregnancy, conflict increases between partners. How are things going with you and your partner as you anticipate the birth of your child?"

In our mobile society, couples may not have family members living close by to educate them about or support them in infant and child care. Confusion about what is normal and abnormal for each stage of child development is common. Therefore, health care providers should make education a part of every sick or well-baby visit and ask how the parents are adjusting.

In American culture, parents are supposed to be positive about parenting. However, the reality is that, along with the joy of parenting, disappointment, frustration, and exhaustion may occur. Individuals who have experienced significant loss or trauma as children may have long-forgotten memories or feelings resurface. Some new parents may not have had positive role models in their own parents. This can make them determined to do well as parents, even to the extent that they demand perfect parenting of themselves. All parents make mistakes and are learning "on the job" to some extent. Health care providers should encourage proper nurturing and caring and give more realistic viewpoints. They can assist new parents in understanding the resilience of children and become valued counselors. Some individuals in couple relationships also are disappointed when the birth or adoption of a child does not solve a marital problem or bring their partner emotionally closer to them. Therefore, child care illustrates the importance of a family-systems approach. Some important educational concepts that can be given to parents are found in Exhibit 2.1.

With the added stress of child care, more conflict may arise in the couple relationship, and less couple time may occur. A decline in marital satisfaction occurs with the transition to parenthood, and it is more pronounced in women (Shapiro et al., 2000). A buffer against the decline of marital satisfaction for a woman is her husband's expression of fondness and admiration for her. Negativity and criticism have been found to be corrosive factors in marital relationships (Sharpiro et al., 2000).

Sexuality and couple time often decline during early parenthood. Parents of small children may have more fantasies about sleep than about intimacy and little time for either.

At times, parents may discuss with their health care providers plans to have additional children. The best advice regarding spacing of children is that there is no "ideal" spacing, and that parents should select an interval that is best for their family situation. Young children have more negative reactions to the birth of a sibling, but regressive behaviors usually dissipate by the end of the first year (Kramer and Ramsburg, 2002). The effectiveness of hospital-based sibling preparation classes is not certain, but they may be a reasonable approach for parents to take.

Some of the stressors for couples with young children include finding child care, dividing household duties, keeping the couple relationship intact, parenting style, and agreeing on the number of children.

EXHIBIT 2.1.
Health Professionals Assisting Patients
with Parenting: Key Concepts

• Normalize the fact that parenting has joys *and* frustrations.
• Assess amount of other stress upon the family, resources of the family for support, and if parent(s) simply needs guidance or if the children appear to be in danger. If children appear to be at risk for harm, immediately refer to proper level of intervention such as family therapist, or contact child protective services (CPS).
• If both parents are in the household, encourage a joint decision to be united on parenting methods, discipline, and encouragement of the children.
• Regarding discipline, lessen expectations for immediate results and gain commitment for staying with a plan for several weeks, even if no initial change in the child's behavior.
• Stress a consistent, nonreactive, reasonable, and age-appropriate approach to discipline that includes time-outs and/or consequences for improper behavior and specific rewards for proper behavior. (The parent(s) should keep emotions in check and refrain from being pulled into arguments with the children.)
• Assist parent(s) in understanding the children's developmental levels.
• Be sure the parent(s) is/are not being overly punitive or expecting the children to have the maturity of an adult.
• Encourage the parent(s) to have a family meeting to discuss what is needed from the children and what the consequences of behaviors will be.
• According to the developmental level of the children, have the parent(s) post, in a prominent place, the main behaviors expected and rewards and consequences.
• Be sure the parent(s) understands the importance of affirmation, praise, and support of good behaviors as well as the value of focused time with children.
• If parent(s) does not appear reasonable, is overly punitive, or if there is intense conflict between the parents, refer them to a family therapist.

THE FAMILY WITH ADOLESCENTS

One individual, who was considered an expert on child care, traveled the country giving a seminar titled "The Ten Commandments for Raising Children." Later, after he had children of his own, he changed the title to "Ten Guidelines for Raising Children," and later to "Ten Suggestions for Raising Children." When his children became teenagers, he stopped giving seminars. Raising children has a way of humbling the best of parents. Some adolescents can be extremely challenging, but most make it through adolescence with no major upheavals.

The physical and emotional adjustments of the adolescent are paralleled by the adjustment in the family system as a whole. This can be a most challenging time for the family as well as a time of emotional growth for the family and adolescent if it is negotiated well. As a child moves into adolescence, family dynamics that have been evolving become more pronounced. If the child has been difficult or parents have not set firm limits, the behavior of the adolescent may erupt into full-blown rebellion. If the family is arrested at an earlier stage of development, such as expecting the adolescent to comply with the rules that were set for a five-year-old child, misunderstandings will occur. The family health care provider, while being careful not to get caught in the middle of the parent-adolescent conflict, can encourage compromise that maintains the safety rules for the adolescent. Assisting parents in seeing that holding on too tightly can lead to more rebellion by the adolescent and assisting the adolescent in avoiding extreme behaviors can be a way of modulating a crisis. Some families need more intensive family therapy during such transitions.

> Patty, a fourteen-year-old girl, is brought by her mother for an office visit for an upper respiratory infection. When alone with you, Patty requests a prescription for oral contraceptives. She does not want her mother to know about her request. The mother is a long-standing patient, and you know that she would not approve of her daughter being prescribed contraceptives.

Health care providers must have a policy on how confidentiality will be ensured and what the exceptions to confidentiality should be (e.g., threat of suicide) when working with adolescents and their parents. The issues of confidentiality and consent are complex, and every family health care provider should be familiar with state laws regarding requests by adolescents for medical care and the confidentiality of their records (see Resources). The Supreme Court of the United States has given adolescents certain rights, such as the right to privacy regarding contraceptives (McDaniel et al., 1990).

Health care providers may have different requirements depending on whether they work in a federally funded clinic or a private practice. Most states give certain minors the right to request medical care concerning pregnancy, substance abuse treatment, contraceptives, and sexually transmitted and contagious diseases. Age limits and the extent of the consent and confidentiality vary. Many awkward situations can be prevented by communicating clearly with parents and adolescents about the rights to and limits of confidentiality and the importance of privacy. Sometimes, when parents must be told certain information, offering the adolescent the opportunity to tell his or her parents with the health care provider present may be helpful. When patients have options about participating in medical decisions, they can gain a better sense of autonomy and control.

Health care providers should continue a therapeutic relationship with both the parents and the adolescent; otherwise, he or she can get caught in the middle. The health care provider should resist the anxiety that many parents bring to the office and avoid their expectation that immediate results should occur. In many of these situations, the problems have been festering for years, so it is unrealistic for parents to expect the health care provider to "fix" everything all at once. Often, developing a plan or some structure for addressing the issues, acting in a nonanxious manner, and truly listening to all parties can lessen the tension in family conflicts (McDaniel et al., 1990).

Once the health care provider's policy on confidentiality is understood, seeing the adolescent alone is important. This communicates to the adolescent that the health care provider values his or her opinions and statements and desires to listen respectfully. Many adolescents want to be able to speak and ask questions in private. Often, they will not reveal this need overtly and may seem apathetic about seeing a health care provider. Finding a balance between engaging them appropriately but not pursuing them to the point where they feel crowded can be a delicate task. Focusing on factual, closed-ended questions may give the adolescent a feeling of safety at the beginning of an office visit (e.g., "What grade are you in?" or "How many years have you lived in this city?"). As the adolescent becomes more comfortable with the health care provider, more open-ended, nonthreatening questions, including some related to areas of interest (e.g., sports and music), can be incorporated. The family health care provider often has the advantage of having established a relationship with the patient in childhood that may endure into adolescence.

Families dealing with the pressures of adolescence often are also dealing with the pressures of grandparents who need care. Parents who are caught between the pressures of caring for their children and caring for their aging parents have been called *the sandwiched generation.* At times, the needs of elderly parents bring long-buried conflicts with parents and siblings to the surface. On the other hand, caregiving of aging parents can have benefits, such as assistance from the parents with finances and household tasks that can reduce caregiver stress. Health care providers can help caregivers belonging to the sandwiched generation by encouraging them to accept assistance from others and helping them realize, use, and enjoy the companionship of their parents (Ingersoll-Dayton et al., 2001).

LAUNCHING CHILDREN AND MOVING ON

Anna and Jim have invested most of their married life in raising their children. The youngest of the three children is leaving for college in the fall. They are excited when they talk with others about the freedom they will have soon. They are both feeling sad, but they have not verbalized these feelings. Anna and Jim also find themselves feeling a lot of uncertainty about the future. Their marriage has been basically good, but it seems that they no longer have much in common. Anna wonders if she might become bored with the marriage and the way Jim always wants to "stay around the house." During an annual health examination, you ask Anna how she is feeling about the so-called "empty nest" that soon will be her experience. In the confidential setting of the office, Anna is able to share her feelings and make statements that she has been barely able to admit to herself. You explain that these feelings are normal and suggest that she and Jim discuss some of the plans they might have, both individually and as a couple. You also give a positive spin to the upcoming transition by saying it is an opportunity for Jim and Anna to reconnect and rediscover good things about their marriage.

This stage of the family life cycle is the period from the time children exit the family until parental retirement. An adolescent leaving home may be the first exit of a family member. Exits and entries can be particularly difficult for families.

If the adolescent has helped in some way to stabilize the parents' marriage, the parents may be fearful about the void created by this exit from the family. The house may seem strange and quiet as the couple adjusts to being alone and to accepting new routines. Some couples find this to be a time of newfound freedom and a period of renewal of activities and social engagements. Some find satisfaction in knowing that the childrearing phase has passed.

Roles change as members exit. If a parent has been a caregiver and his or her primary identity was as a parent, he or she may wonder what his or her role will be now that the child has left. Encouraging parents to try new things, such as going back to school or taking up a new hobby, may be important to moving them in a positive direction.

Some individuals have reached the peak of their careers and have no additional career goals to achieve. Others find themselves being let go by their employers and having to seek new positions during middle age while competing with younger workers. This can put tremendous strain on a couple's relationship. Feelings of anger, rejection, and loss can carry over into the marriage and create distance between partners.

During this phase of the family life cycle, new members may be added to the extended family system. Children attach to mates and begin their own families. If the parents do not approve of their child's choice of a mate, another source of stress is created. Expectations may be too great, and some parents may want their children to marry someone who is similar to their own spouse; issues about socioeconomic, religious, cultural, racial, and educational differences also can cause conflict.

THE FAMILY IN LATER LIFE

A rapidly growing segment of the population is in this stage of family life and will spend more time in this period because of increased longevity. This stage often is associated with several losses, including the couple experiencing the loss of their parents, which brings emotional stress and the realization of their own mortality. Generational roles shift, and they become the matriarch and patriarch of the family. Where they may have once relied on the counsel of their parents, they now may be bereft without this source of support. The couple now may assume this role for the younger generations.

Retirement may be a difficult adjustment for the individual and the couple. Work provides structure for much of an individual's time and provides social and financial benefits. When life has been centered primarily on work, the transition to retirement becomes more intense. In addition, some couples function well with the distance created by careers, and a sudden increase in time spent together may strain the relationship.

Other losses include the loss of friends due to death or relocation, and the individual's own failing health and loss of function and ability for self-care. The loss of a longtime companion is one of the most painful life events. When a partner or friend dies, it is hard to replace the continuity of these long histories that an individual has developed over a lifetime. Many elderly individuals begin a precipitous decline in health as losses begin to multiply.

The approach to the end of life can, of course, be difficult for families, couples, and individuals. We all carry a certain denial with us about loss and the end of life. Herbert Anderson (1999) wrote: "We need to understand that all of life is framed by birth and death. *And we are most likely to discover the deeper truth about human finitude through a spiritual pilgrimage rather than a psychological exploration*" (p. 170). Erik Erikson (1993) termed the stage of late adulthood as one of ego integrity versus ego despair and this depicts the issues that many face in later life as they come to terms with the history of their lives and the losses and changes that are occurring. For some families and individual family members the later stage of life can precipitate a spiritual or existential crisis as adaptations to life and life meanings can occur in rapid-fire manner. Figure 2.1 diagrams possible pathways to spiritual crisis which may occur at any stage of life, but certainly have several components that occur frequently in later life. Perhaps those who tend to move toward and through later life with greater

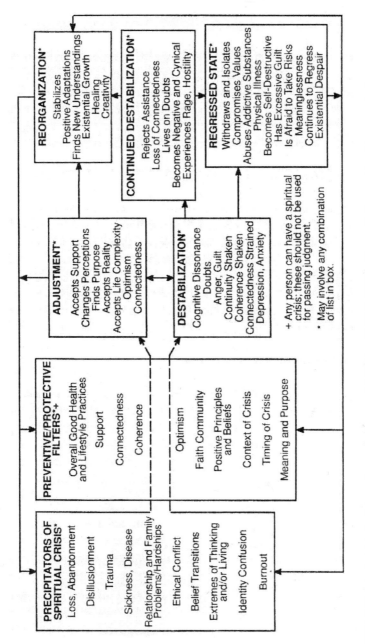

FIGURE 2.1. Spiritual crisis pathways. *Source:* McBride. 1998:5. © The Haworth Press. Used by permission.

27

ease have incorporated more or have access to more preventive and protective filters such as overall good health practices, family and friendship support, and ways of finding meaning and purpose in life.

Before the emergence of a health or other life crisis, the family health care provider can give anticipatory guidance, encourage the development of support systems, plan for care at an assisted living or nursing home facility, and discuss desires in terms of a living will. Some individuals have great difficulty adjusting to becoming dependent on others for their care. Health care providers should provide opportunities for elderly patients to express their emotions in this regard. Encouraging family members and other caregivers to allow as much independence as possible is essential.

The rate of completed suicide is high in the elderly. Widowed white men have an especially high rate of suicide and should be assessed for depression and suicidal ideation. Most elderly individuals who complete a suicide will have visited their primary care health care provider in the weeks preceding the suicide. However, suicidal thoughts most often are not discussed unless the health care provider asks about them. Health care providers should inquire about any thoughts of self-harm if the patient has experienced a loss or has any indication of depression.

Chapter 3

Variations to the Family Life Cycle

Most families' experiences do not follow the concise structure of the family life cycle that has been described. Many events can change or alter the family life cycle. Divorce, death of children, single or childless adults, same-sex couples, and blended families are a few factors that can cause the family life cycle to vary.

BLENDED FAMILIES

Couples and families separate for a variety of reasons and rejoin in a variety of forms, stretching and expanding the concept and definition of family. Understanding the reorganization and adaptation that is required of the remarried or blended family is essential. The complexity of relationships, alliances, boundaries, and loyalties can be extensive when previously married individuals with children remarry.

Important data regarding the remarried family culled from the literature by McGoldrick and Carter (1999, pp. 417-422) include the following:

1. Stepfamilies are becoming the most common family form.
2. Women with higher levels of education and income are less likely to remarry; the opposite is true for men.
3. Couples with stepchildren are twice as likely to divorce—approximately one fourth divorce within the first five years.
4. Finances are often a major problem in remarried families.

Family Behavioral Issues in Health and Illness
Published by The Haworth Press, Inc., 2006. All rights reserved.
doi:10.1300/5621_03

Remarriage and rejoining may be just as momentous as the first marriage or cohabitation. Just as some individuals have unrealistic ideas about first marriages, some also have idealistic and unrealistic ideas about remarriage and enter the union not realizing the work that will be required. Parents and children may still be grieving the loss of the previous family structure. The new partners often already have children, so the couple may not have an opportunity to bond by themselves.

The health care provider can assist by explaining how such changes are normal and urging lower expectations of immediate resolution of all issues. Roles, rules, and relationships are all in flux and will need time to settle into comfortable positions. Emphasizing the importance of flexibility and accommodation can be an important component of anticipatory guidance. Often, stepparents want to assume the parental and disciplinarian roles with stepchildren as soon as the marriage occurs. This usually does not work and can create a rebellious reaction in adolescents. Counseling parents to not push too hard with their stepchildren and encouraging the biological parent to be in charge of the discipline can assist with lessening conflict. Allowing a friendship to develop and appropriate bonding to occur between stepparents and stepchildren must be the foundation upon which active parenting eventually is built, and this can take two years or more (Visher and Visher, 1996). A common adjustment in the remarried family is a feeling by children or a spouse that their needs are being ignored and that more energy is being spent on another family member.

In summary, the health care provider can assist by offering basic counseling to patients contemplating remarriage or those in a new remarriage by emphasizing the work that will need to be done, the flexibility that will be necessary, and the patience required to allow relationships to evolve over time. Because of the complexity and the number of individuals involved, referral to a family therapist should be considered as an option before conflict becomes ingrained or unmanageable.

SINGLE-PARENT FAMILIES

The number of children living with single parents has approximately doubled since 1970 to 31 percent in 2000. These families are often the result of teenage or adult pregnancies in unmarried women, divorce, parental death, adoption, or parental separation.

From the start, many of these families are in a difficult financial position. Only one income is supporting the family, and most single parents are women who traditionally have worked for lower wages than men. A higher percentage of children from single-parent homes have problems, such as academic and behavioral difficulties (Meurer et al., 1996). The emotional, physical, and financial overload can limit time for a parent's personal life and leave the parent more vulnerable to additional stressors. Often the single parent is in a position of role strain, attempting to balance a job with family responsibilities. However, most of the problems for children in single-parent households are the same as those for children in two-parent households.

In reality, some single-parent families function well with the support of extended family members. Involvement with groups, such as community agencies and religious organizations that can offer support, may be vital for some single-parent families. More resources are needed for these families because many single parents do not have extended family members to assist them.

A potential danger in the single-parent family is for a parent to depend too heavily on a child and begin to place the child into a peer-like role. This is called a *loss of intergenerational boundaries*. For example, a divorced parent might need the emotional support of a child and, consequently, share personal feelings that overburden the child. The child may be pulled out of the sibling subsystem and into a parentified child role, thereby losing the role as a child. This can create conflict or rejection of this child by the other children and be a factor in depressive features in him or her.

In the past, much of the emphasis on single-parent families has been on families with single mothers; however, families with single fathers are increasing. Although single-father families are still a small proportion of all families, the rate of growth has been rapid since 1980, making this one of the fastest-growing family types. Differences have occurred in the demographic profile of these families in the past decade as well. For example, single fathers are likely to have never been married, have younger children with fewer siblings, and be less financially well-off (Eggebeen and Snyder, 1996).

Health care providers can affirm the efforts of single parents and direct them toward supportive networks for themselves and their children. Support may come from extended family members, social agencies, religious institutions, or a combination of these. Also, assessing and, if needed, treating the single parent for depression and burnout is important.

Single-parent families may have more difficulty when children grow up and leave the home. Because some single parents have put their lives on hold in many ways and focused on their children, the void can be felt intensely when the children leave. This is another critical transition point where the parent may need encouragement and direction from the health care provider.

GAY AND LESBIAN FAMILIES

Gay and lesbian couples and families have much in common with heterosexual couples and families, but may also have the additional stressors of being in a society where they have limited acceptance. They may not be open about their lifestyles for fear of a negative effect on their lives, families, and careers. Homophobia, a strong irrational fear of individuals who have or want same-sex unions, continues to be an issue, resulting in prejudice, discrimination, and even severe violence. Viewing the entire family relationship in terms of sexuality may negate or cause other areas of a couple's relationship to be ignored (Harrison, 1996).

Health care providers can help families confronting such problems by helping them recognize how these problems can affect the overall functioning of the family. Community involvement and support may be limited. Extended family members may reject the family when sexual orientation is revealed. This forced isolation can place increased pressure on gay or lesbian families and increase the risk for substance abuse, depression, suicide attempts, and anxiety. Those with couple or family problems may have few outside resources for assistance. They may delay or avoid seeking health care because of fear of discrimination and stigmatization (Clark et al., 2001).

Gay and lesbian couple relationships tend to be more egalitarian than heterosexual relationships, with more shared decision-making responsibility. Gender role socialization affects gay and lesbian relationships. Lesbian relationships have been found to value emotional expressiveness and nurturing, which is in keeping with female socialization in our society. Gay relationships are characterized by more frequent and varied sexual activities, which can be linked with heterosexual male socialization. Coming from a stable family of origin and having a history of good psychosocial functioning is more important to and predictive of positive family relationships than whether one is heterosexual or homosexual (Glick et al., 2000).

No systematic differences exist in emotional health, parenting skills, and attitudes toward parenting between gay and lesbian and nongay and nonlesbian parents (Perrin, 2002). According to the American Association of Pediatrics (2002),

> The American Academy of Pediatrics recognizes that a considerable body of professional literature provides evidence that children with parents who are homosexual can have the same advantages and the same expectations for health, adjustment, and development as can children whose parents are heterosexual. (p. 339)

This statement was made, in part, to encourage protection of the rights of children to maintain continuing relationships with both their biological parents and their co-parents in same-sex unions. The American Academy of Family Physicians' Congress of Delegates also authored a position and policy statement for children and adoptive parents in October 2002 that aims to "be supportive of legislation, which promotes a safe and nurturing environment, including psychological and legal security, for all children, including those of adoptive parents, regardless of the parents' sexual orientation."

AIDS has had a significant effect on the gay community, resulting in the loss of multiple friends, intensified anxiety, and increased stigma for members of the gay community. Even with the progress in the treatment of human immunodeficiency virus (HIV) infection, evidence suggests that high-risk behavior may now be on the rise possibly because of a false sense of security among some individuals who believe that HIV is a manageable chronic condition (Gay and Lesbian Medical Association, 2001).

Extended family members may first learn about an individual's sexual orientation when he or she is diagnosed with AIDS. In these situations, the patient and family have the double task of adjusting to the news about the sexual orientation and dealing with the profound effects of the infection. Patients and families may need education and support during this time.

Lesbian, gay, and bisexual adolescent patients who reside in or are from heterosexual families often experience family conflict or even physical abuse because of their sexual orientation. Gay, lesbian, and bisexual adolescents are at increased risk for depression, suicide attempts, and substance abuse (Cope, 2001).

Health care professionals should assess how intake forms, health care provider history-taking and interviewing processes, and language can reveal biases toward some groups. Regardless of a professional's personal beliefs, all patients should have access to complete, confidential, and nonjudgmental health care (see Resources).

FAMILIES WITH INFERTILITY

Frequently, couples need support in dealing with infertility. Allowing them the opportunity to express emotions about accepting infertility is important. For those who desire children, a diagnosis of infertility can be a major adjustment. For example, a recent randomized study found that infertility was associated with statistically significant long-term psychological distress and threatened a central life identity for women who never had children (McQuillan et al., 2003). Anticipatory guidance about treatment options and the possible emotional and relationship responses are important. Infertility can affect the individuals personally and the couple's relationships in numerous ways. On a personal level, issues of self-esteem and role identity as well as frustration, disappointment, and depression may arise. Fertility tests and procedures can become intrusive and take away some of the spontaneity from sexual relations.

Some couples weather the process well, but others become overly focused on the infertility or the treatment success or failure. Emphasis should be placed on the couple's relationship and not entirely on the diagnosis and treatment issues (Whitman-Elia and Baxley, 2001).

ADOPTIVE FAMILIES

Adoptive families have different challenges, including the following:

1. Acknowledgment of difference (refers to the way the family acknowledges the uniqueness of being an adoptive rather than a biological family)
2. The parents' sense of control over the extent to which the child's birth family members are included in their family life
3. Entitlement (the parents' sense of their right to be the child's full parents)
4. Loss (refers to the loss experienced by all parties—the adoptive parents' possible loss of fertility, the child's loss of his or her birth family, the birth parents' loss of the child)
5. Adoptive identity (the adolescent's emerging sense of self as an adopted individual)
6. Perceived compatibility (refers to the compatibility with the adoptive family as sensed by the child) (Miller et al., 2000, p. 1509)

Because of the scarcity of newborns available for adoption, the number of private adoptions, international adoptions, and adoptions of children with special needs has increased (Sherry and Nickman, 1999; Gavagan and Brodyaga, 1998; Quarles and Brodie, 1998). These children and their families may have special medical and emotional needs. Assisting the adoptive parents in understanding any medical conditions the child may have is extremely important. The parents need as realistic a picture as possible about any additional demands the child may make on them. Parents who are too idealistic and do not consider all factors can become disillusioned and discouraged. Parents may also need support when they are going through a possibly intrusive adoption screening process.

Some children of multiethnic adoptions have difficulty with identity development, which can be complicated by behavioral and learning problems, educational deficits, and trauma histories (Friedlander, 1999). International adoptees may have little opportunity to interact with individuals from their native countries. Helping multiethnic adoptive families see that many of their challenges are due to cultural transition and adjustment can lessen the sense of dysfunction among members.

All children should be told in a caring and loving way that they are adopted. Some adoption experts believe the process should begin when the child is between the ages of two and four, while others encourage openness from the beginning. Similar to sex education, the health care provider should assist the parents in discussing adoption with their child in a way that is developmentally appropriate. Adoptive parents may need affirmation that they are parenting correctly. The health care provider can assist with basic parenting techniques and offer assurances.

If an older adopted child wants to contact his or her birth parents, the family health care provider can assist the adoptive parent with accepting this as a normal phase in the development of many adoptees (see Resources).

FAMILIES WITHOUT CHILDREN

Couples who do not have children are often misunderstood in our society. They do not have some of the life experiences of couples with children. When counseling infertile couples, health care providers should include the option to not have children rather than undergoing fertility procedures. Health care providers must be careful about stating assumptions, such as "when you have kids," which would be more appropriately stated as "if you have kids." Common expressions, such as "Who will take care of you in old age?" and "You are too young to have surgical sterilization," can reveal paternalistic biases of the health care provider. Couples making decisions about having children need a nonjudgmental approach that gives them the medical information necessary to make clear decisions and that communicates the freedom and right of the couple to choose what is best for their family situation.

Currently, support structures are largely lacking for childless couples. Health care providers should be sensitive to the issues of these couples and offer permission to discuss their feelings and concerns openly. Voluntary childlessness has increased in recent decades, while involuntary childlessness has declined because of better health and less sterility caused by sexually transmitted diseases (Heaton et al., 1999). In the last decade, the expectation that all married couples should have children and that the main purpose of marriage is to have children has decreased (Thorton and Young-DeMarco, 2001) (see Resources).

FAMILIES FROM OTHER CULTURES

Awareness about the diversity in family life in the United States has grown. Generalizations made about families based on studies of American samples may not be valid in other cultural contexts (Parke, 2000). The following summary of a case presented in the literature, although from ethnographic interviews rather than medical interviews, illustrates well the importance of cultural understanding. When health care providers are dealing with a particular cultural population, it is imperative to develop a reasonable understanding of how symptoms, explanatory models of illness, family involvement in treatment, and treatments and remedies are understood within that culture.

Tran, a Vietnamese woman, immigrated to Canada. She had numerous somatic and emotional symptoms with no medical explanation. She believed that her symptoms were from the weakness or loss of energy (qi) that she, after a long interview, linked to an experience in Vietnam. She had fallen in love with a married man and had an affair. To preserve her family's honor, she left Vietnam. However, she missed the relationship with the man and was very lonely. She explained that her depression was related to the injustice of being accused of being a bad daughter while she believed her feelings for her lover were noble. She had seen a practitioner of traditional Vietnamese medicine who gave her remedies to treat her weakness, but Tran did not tell him her secret. She could not speak to anyone about the affair or its consequences out of respect for her family's reputation and the reputation of her lover's family.

Because the ethnographic interviewer was not Vietnamese and was not a threat to her family's honor or her social position, Tran was able to tell her secret and begin to feel better. She was no longer pessimistic about her future and even progressed to the point of wanting to find a psychotherapist to assist her (Kirmayer and Groleau, 2001).

Even with good intrafamily support, immigration can be stressful. Because of the effect on and adjustment of the entire family, a family-systems approach is the more effective intervention. Examining health care in the context of cultural and social backgrounds is important. Health belief systems and explanatory models of illness must be assessed. Historical data, such as the circumstances of immigration, the length of time in the United States, and what the experience has been like, are important (Slonim-Nevo, Sharaga, and Mirsky, 1999). Did the family view the United States with great idealism only to be disappointed by the prejudice they experienced? What losses have been associated with the move? Are other family members still in the county of origin? At what age or point in the life cycle did the individual or family emigrate? Questions such as these can assist the health care provider in assessing the historical dynamics of the family and its influence on health and future health care.

Refugees, in particular, should be assessed for anxiety, depression, physical abuse, substance abuse, and post-traumatic stress disorder (PTSD) (Gavagan and Brodyaga, 1998). Most refugees have a sponsoring agency that assists in the resettlement process and can be a resource for the family health care provider (Kang et al., 1998). Refugees often are isolated, have significant stressors, and lack resources. The potential for family problems can be high. A family health care provider may be one of the few individuals with the potential to intervene by assessing the family dynamics and potential for danger within the family.

Sensitivity to the variety of ways families from various cultures conduct family life and relations is important. There may be greater distance or closeness among members, greater authority given to parents or children, differing parenting styles, variations in gender roles, and different understandings about the roles of health care providers and patients compared with the cultural norms of the health care provider. Genuine openness, interest, and curiosity as a means of clarification can be well accepted by those individuals from other cultures.

INTERGENERATIONAL FAMILIES

The grandparent role in America has become more complex because of changing family structures and longevity (some families consist of three, four, and five generations) (Mills, 2001). Grandparent caregiving is more prevalent in black families (approximately 29 percent of grandmothers and 14 percent of grandfathers serve as surrogate parents to their grandchildren) than in white or Hispanic families in the United States (Fuller-Thomson and Minkeler, 2000). In approximately 3.2 million households, grandparents are raising grandchildren as the result of informal arrangements, legal arrangements, or interventions by the child welfare system (Kelley and Damato, 1996).

This can be a rewarding arrangement for a grandparent and child, but it can also place difficult strains on the individuals involved. Grandparents may be in a difficult financial situation or have failing health. In some cases, grandparents assuming the parenting role for grandchildren results from the death of parents or from parents being deemed unfit to care for the children. Such families are at greater risk for problems. Additional potential issues include challenges or difficulties within the relationship between the parents and the grandparents and between the child and the parents. Support from other family members or community resources may be needed (see Resources).

MULTIRACIAL AND MULTIETHNIC FAMILIES

In 1967, the Supreme Court of the United States declared laws unconstitutional that prohibited interracial marriages. Since then, the number of interracial marriages has increased gradually. Social and cultural mores have continued to discourage interracial marriages in many areas. Among black and white married individuals, nonracial homogenous factors or perceived social similarities, such as common interests and personal attractiveness, have been found to be more important than racial issues in spouse selection (Lewis et al., 1997).

Much of the theory on interracial coupling developed in the 1960s and 1970s was based on psychologic myths, such as "black sexual acting out," "white neurotic acting out," and the psychologic shortcomings of interracial children. A new model developed for multiracial couples includes the stages of racial awareness, coping, identity emergence, and relationship maintenance (Foeman and Nance, 1999). For example, these couples must learn, along with other coupling issues, their partner's collective racial group's perspective, cope with intolerant reactions of others, and develop skills needed in a multicultural society.

Little research has been done on multiracial and multiethnic children and their families. Until the 2000 census, government census data did not allow for identification of individuals as multiracial. On birth certificates, children traditionally have been recorded according to the mother's race or ethnicity, making such research impossible. Because of several factors, including an environment that does not appreciate diversity, racial identity development can be a difficult and complex process for some biracial children, especially during adolescence. Health care providers should be sensitive to at-risk behaviors, such as depression, poor school performance, negative attitudes about adults, social isolation, "chip on the shoulder" attitudes, psychosomatic disorders, and suicidal ideation, that can occur in biracial youth as they move toward integration and appreciation of all the backgrounds they possess (Benedetto and Olisky, 2001; Nishimura, 1995).

Chapter 4

Special Family Topics

DIVORCE

Although the nurse has noted a lingering headache as the reason for the office visit, you know as soon as you walk into the examining room that something traumatic is going on with Tina, who has been a patient for several years. As you close the door, Tina can no longer maintain control and begins shaking and sobbing. Initially unable to speak, she gradually is able to talk in short phrases interrupted by emotional heaves and tears. She relates that her husband has told her that their seven-year marriage is over. He told her this in a rather matter-of-fact manner and did not appear to be sensitive to her feelings. She is shocked. Tina knows that since the birth of their first child five years ago and, especially, since the birth of their second child three years later, that her main focus has been on the children. Her husband, John, appeared to be consumed with his career. Tina also worked outside the home and did more than her share of the housework and child care. John did not give Tina any options, and he stated that his decision was not impulsive and that he had been considering it for some time.

Tina had never considered that the relationship might end. She is at a loss about what to do. She does not have the money to see a counselor and does not want to see one. You listen to her and acknowledge the emotional pain and distress that she is experiencing by using statements such as, "Tina, I know this is very traumatic for you and has turned your world upside down. It will take some time to sort it all out." Later in the visit, you state, "Let's come up with a basic structure of things you can do, such as seeing your rabbi and coming regularly to see me, as you adjust." You know she is active in a local temple and encourage her to ask for a private meeting with her rabbi. Over the next few months, you have Tina schedule regular follow-up visits during which you normalize many of the intense feelings she shares and encourage her to maintain a healthy lifestyle of exercise and social interactions. Tina experiences depression, but not to the extent that she needs antidepressants. You feel

Family Behavioral Issues in Health and Illness
Published by The Haworth Press, Inc., 2006. All rights reserved.
doi:10.1300/5621_04

that you have assisted her in making the adjustment with your simple ac-knowledgments of her feelings and basic interventions, yet you did not fall into the trap of dictating what she should do or condemning her spouse during the divorce process. Tina's rabbi, who had formal training in counseling, intervened with more of the family dynamics.

Although divorce is not as socially stigmatizing as it was a few decades ago, it can still send shock waves through the family system, especially if the extended family has not been aware of the marital problems or if there have been no prior divorces in the family. Religious beliefs and church doctrines also can be factors in adjusting to news of a divorce. Broken relationships with the former spouse's extended family also may occur. On the other hand, some couples, children, and extended family systems appear to adjust to divorce without a major upheaval.

The divorcing partners may react to divorce in a variety of ways. One spouse may have been unaware of the other partner's movement toward divorce until the actual news is given or a crisis (e.g., an affair) becomes known. The partner seeking the divorce already may have progressed past the point of grieving for the marriage and feel ready to move on, while the other partner may be just entering the grieving stage of the marital dissolution. Roles may reverse at times during the divorce process, with one partner wanting out and the other hanging on. Then, the opposite occurs. Men initially may appear to be making a better emotional adjustment than women, but this often is reversed at some point after the divorce.

The divorce process may be permeated with ambivalence. One day, the divorced person may feel that he or she cannot survive and the next may feel that he or she is "over" the ex-spouse. The person may move from elation to depression in just a few hours. Thus, the divorce process has appropriately been called a "crazy time" by some. Anticipating this emotional roller-coaster ride with patients and sharing the normalcy of it is important. Otherwise, they may feel they are losing all control of their lives. Individuals can find themselves behaving out of character under the stress of divorce.

Extramarital affairs can be particularly devastating to a marriage and may generate a severe crisis for the spouse who has been betrayed. Obsessing about the details of the extramarital affair and ambivalence about the continuation of the marriage usually occur. The patient in such a situation should be assessed for depression, anxiety, and homicidal and suicidal ideation. Often, the individual is so agitated that it is difficult for him or her to eat or sleep. Trust is often shattered as well as basic assumptions about the marriage and, possibly, even about life itself. Some are so angry that they are ready to end the marriage immediately. Others overfunction in pursuing their spouses in an attempt to win them back.

The health care provider can assist by encouraging the slowing of intense reactivity and suggesting that the partner attempt to be firm about his or her conditions for the marriage continuing without constantly pursuing or raging at the partner. Health care providers also can discourage rash decision making, offer emotional support, provide opportunities for ventilation, and make referrals for marital therapy. The health care provider must be careful about what he or she says about the partner who is involved in the affair. The health care provider should not get too involved in the emotional field of the marital problems. Although not affirming the affair, the larger context and the other spouse's story might give a very different picture of the marital dynamics. The old adage, "there are two sides to every story," is important for the health care provider to keep in mind. The concepts included in Exhibit 4.1 should be considered when working with divorcing patients.

After a divorce, some individuals rush into another relationship or marriage as a means of escaping from emotional pain. This can result in delaying the grieving process and prematurely establishing a new family. Often there is a "transitional relationship" that will not survive but serves as a conduit to move the individual on with life. Sometimes family members and friends pressure the divorced individual to start dating before he or she feels ready and may set up blind dates or "chance" meetings of potential partners. The divorced individual must set some limits and not allow himself or herself to be coerced into situations for which he or she is not ready or interested.

In many areas of the country, individuals trained as divorce mediators act as a neutral party to negotiate a settlement. Mediation has been shown to reduce the intense conflict and legal battles that often are associated with divorce and may even contribute to the

EXHIBIT 4.1.
Health Professionals Assisting Patients
in Relationship Distress

- *Keep alert to relationship problems.* Vague somatic complaints may indicate relationship distress. Ask about family and relationships: "How are things going at home?" "How are things in your relationship (marriage)?"
- *Express empathy.* Communicate a sense of how his or her world has been "turned upside down," or use another phrase that expresses that the emotional pain is difficult, when the patient shares intense distress over a relationship.
- *Allow ventilation.* Do not stifle strong feelings and normalize that these are usual for persons in relationship distress. The patient may feel there is something wrong with him or her because of the intensity of the feelings. The physician may want to encourage the patient to write about feelings in a confidential journal.
- *Assess commitment to relationship.* Is there any commitment left to work on the relationship? Some have already made a firm decision to end the relationship, others have an impulse to end the relationship, but underneath the reactivity they want the relationship to continue. Ask: "Have you made a final decision to end the relationship or are you willing to work on saving it?"
- *Slow down impulsivity.* Even if the patient has decided to end the relationship, unless there is danger such as domestic violence, it may be appropriate to ask, "What's the rush?" if he or she is impulsively wanting to end the relationship. Often such major decisions do not need to be rushed and the physician can assist in helping the person slow down the process and carefully look at all sides of the issues.
- *Refrain from being the authority on the patient's relationship.* The physician should guard against telling the patient to ultimately leave the relationship or stay in it. The decision needs to be made by the patient.
- *Educate.* Convey concepts that all long-term relationships can go through various phases and take a lot of work and energy to be rewarding.
- *Help contain fallout.* Assist the person in the containment of the negatives about the partner. He or she is vulnerable to telling everyone everything and then regretting it if he or she remains in the relationship. Suggest that discussion of all the details should be limited to a few trusted friends, clergy, or other professionals.

- *Encourage structure.* In the midst of the chaos that relationship breakups entail, exercise, eating properly, being active, and keeping a schedule can help.
- *Be cautious with comments about patient's partner.* The physician should be careful not to make negative comments about the partner. It may be that the patient will be on good terms with his or her partner next week and remember the negative statements the physician made about the person he or she loves!
- *Direct from partner focus to self-focus.* As the person stabilizes, encourage self-focus on what the patient could do to enhance the relationship. "You have only mentioned several things you want your partner to change. I am wondering what things you have decided you will do to help the relationship?"
- *Assess risk.* Check for suicidal and homicidal ideation or intent and potential for domestic violence.
- *Evaluate need for medication.* Consider psychotropic medication as appropriate.
- *Set up follow-up appointments.* Give the patient the structure of regular appointments for the near future and include the partner soon if restoring the relationship is a goal for the couple.
- *Refer if necessary.* Refer to a counselor if longstanding conflicts and defensiveness have existed in the relationship, the patient does not respond to primary care intervention in a few weeks, or if there is risk of suicide, homicide, or violence.

safety of the female spouse (Ellis, 2000). This can be an asset to the divorce adjustment process and aid in moving the individuals in a healthy direction. Divorce mediation may be less likely to succeed if both partners are fixated on winning over the other or if an extreme power imbalance is evident in the relationship.

Most divorced individuals remarry within a few years. Ideally, remarriage will be entered with more realistic expectations than the first marriage, but many do not appear to learn from the past. In fact, the divorce rate for second marriages is higher than that for first marriages. Some individuals' feelings of loss return when an ex-spouse marries because they see hope of reconciliation of the marriage gone. Others may see it as a sign that the ex-spouse has moved on in a positive direction while their own life is stuck. Support and permission for ventilation of feelings may be important during this time.

Divorce is often seen by professionals in the family field as another stage of life that has become characteristic of our culture. Most individuals faced with divorce initially see it as a crisis and then stabilize after about a year.

Health care providers may be asked how divorce will affect children. Some of the factors that influence a child's adjustment to divorce include the following:

1. The level of interparental conflict that precedes and follows the divorce
2. The number of stressful life events that accompany and follow the divorce
3. The custodial parent's psychologic adjustment and parenting skills
4. The amount and quality of contact with the noncustodial parent
5. The degree of economic hardship to which the children are exposed (Amato, 1994, pp. 150-151; Meurer et al., 1996, p. 867)

The importance of conveying the continued love of both parents for the children and that the children are not the reason for the divorce must be stressed to parents during a divorce process. Providing structure for children during and after the divorce is also important. For example, ensuring that children have some space and items of their own at each parent's home and allowing children to continue in the same schools can minimize the disruption of children's lives.

ABUSE

One of the most difficult aspects of family life to accept is that many persons are victims of abuse by their own family members. Our culture tends to think of the family as a safe haven of acceptance, love, and support, but this is not a reality in some families. Others may have a mixture of support and violence or abuse that can be particularly distressing and confusing. Past tendencies were to view the family as a private arena where government agencies should not intervene even in cases of violence. More communities are now establishing better protocols not only for intervention in child abuse but also spousal abuse. Some communities have shelters such as battered women's shelters that not only offer safe housing for women and their children but also education on family violence. Often cycles of abuse continue through generations of family life unless there is intervention.

Other works address abuse and violence in families in greater detail. Here we will briefly address child abuse, spouse abuse, and elder abuse in the family.

Child Abuse

Professionals who know of or suspect child physical or sexual abuse or neglect of a child are required by law to report it to the proper authorities, usually the department of family and children's services. The primary consideration is the safety and protection of the child. Although abuse of children can occur across all strata of society, some parents who abuse their children have expectations that are too high of their children and may believe their children are the cause of their own problems. Often there is a lack of generational boundaries and lack of parenting skills.

Far too often abusive families are polyabusive and may abuse physically, sexually, and emotionally. The children receive very conflicting messages in such families and often get a strong message that their own needs are not important or valued. Boundaries are violated with the intrusion confusing the self-identity of the children. Such abused children may continue to have problems with limit setting, boundary maintenance, depression, anxiety, and relationship difficulty in adult life. Children who are abused often suffer from shame and guilt and blame themselves for the abuse.

A significant percentage of those who abuse children were abused themselves, but this is by no means always true. At the current level of knowledge we cannot make absolute predictions regarding who will become a child abuser. In addition, it appears that children who are perhaps more difficult to care for or raise (for example, those with a disability) are abused more frequently. This should not be seen as a reason to blame the children, but as a factor in the combination of family stress, lack of proper parenting ability, and poor parental self-control. Family stress has often been linked to child abuse; therefore, assisting the family with finding additional resources, support, and parent education is often one of the most important interventions.

Important issues should be considered when taking a patient history in child and adolescent sexual abuse and important legal and psychological mistakes can be made unless the treating professional has some training or education in this area. In many cases, an expert in interviewing children from an agency such as community child protective services should supplement the work of the health care provider.

Spouse Abuse

The reality of spousal abuse has captivated the media and our attention frequently in recent years. The great majority of cases involve a man abusing his partner or spouse. Issues involved are complicated but involve sexism, control, and power. A cycle of abuse may proceed from a stress and tension-building phase where the woman is accused of various issues such as having an affair and where her self-esteem is attacked. She may live in a very unpredictable environment, not knowing what may bring forth outbursts of anger. This escalates to the actual abuse and violence that can take many forms. Afterward, there is often a phase where the man is repentant and sorry for the abuse. He may apologize or he may become very tender and caring. He often makes promises that he will change and never abuse again. This bonding phase is one reason the partner often finds it difficult to leave the relationship.

Patients accompanied by a partner, especially an overly attentive, demanding, or aggressive partner, should be interviewed alone. The health care provider should simply ask the partner to please go to the waiting room so that the exam can be completed. The health care provider should ask questions about abuse on a routine basis such as, "Many people are exposed to violence in our society. Have you ever been in a relationship where you have been threatened or hurt by your partner?" Should the patient share about abuse, it is essential to convey nonjudgmental acceptance of her story and document by quoting her own words. Materials from resources in the community should be available and, if desired, an opportunity for her to make a private phone call to such resources or protective authorities from the health care provider's office. If she takes any material with her, she should be warned to conceal it in a place where the batterer will not find it since such could increase his anger. One must guard against attempting to impose a time frame for leaving a relationship since this is the decision of the adult involved, who may, in fact, never leave. For the person being battered, deciding to leave can be one of the most difficult of decisions as well as one of the most dangerous. Also, one must be careful not to get frustrated when the battered spouse states she is going to leave and does not or leaves and goes back. The relationship dynamics are complex and a professional with a simplistic view may end up blaming the victim.

One of the best interventions by health care providers in partner abuse is simply listening in a concerned manner and affirming that the victim has options of support in the community and connecting the patient with shelters for the abused and legal authorities. Usually abuse shelters have educational programs or group support meetings as well as a safe place to stay. Another important intervention is having the patient develop an emergency or safety plan of what steps will be taken in the event of abuse or threat to life. Emergency resources such as a place to go in the middle of the night, having important documents readily available such as her driver's license, birth certificates for her and her children, and having some money put away for a crisis is an important part of a plan. Access to needed medications may also be essential.

Also, the time of greatest risk for being killed by an abuser is when the women chooses to leave, so protective measures (e.g., legal restraints or protective orders, and time at a safe shelter) may need to be in place at that time and afterward. A significant percent of couples who experience physical abuse also experience substance abuse, which can complicate risk assessment. For dually affected couples, the substance abuse will also need to be addressed in treatment (Bostock and Auster, 2002).

When considering referral for treatment, recognize that some forms of treatment could escalate the violence. Many believe that treatment for the abuser, especially group therapy, must occur in many cases before family therapy is a safe modality of treatment. A special concern in spousal abuse is the impact it has on children who are observers of the abuse. Too often it is forgotten that these traumatized children are also victims of the abuse.

Elder Abuse

Another group in our society at risk for abuse is the elderly. Elder abuse may involve neglect, being denied food and medications, forced isolation, threats, misuse of financial resources, psychological abuse such as intimidation, and various forms of physical abuse. Again, females are the ones most often abused, but it can occur to either gender. Elderly persons who are dependent and are difficult to care for are more frequent victims. Caregiver stress and frustration is associated with the abuse of elders as well. Sometimes a person abused as a child will abuse the parent in a type of role reversal as the parent ages. Known or suspected elder abuse should be reported to the proper authorities. Many communities now have adult protective services to intervene in such situations. However, often communities do not have adequate resources to address this issue as completely as it should be. In addition, as with spouse abuse, unless the elderly person is mentally incapacitated, he or she has the legal right to choose to remain in the setting where the abuse occurred.

Abuse and Physical Illness

The link between physical and sexual abuse and physical illnesses is realized with various bodily symptoms and increased medical utilization occurring with such patients (Grilo and Masheb, 2001; Stein and Barrett-Connor, 2000). Depression, anxiety disorders, dissociative disorders, PTSD, substance abuse, and eating disorders are among the at-risk disorders in such patients (Grilo and Masheb, 2001; Stein and Barrett-Connor, 2000; Bulick et al., 2001).

Abuse and Spirtuality

An intense impact may be made upon the basic life assumptions and spirituality of persons who experience horrific abuse and trauma (Janoff-Bulman, 1992). This may lead to a shattering of beliefs, profound spiritual questioning, breaking of bonds and connections with others, and distrust of God or others (Hermon, 1992; Sinclair, 1993; McBride and Armstrong, 1995).

MEDICAL ISSUES AND FAMILY LIFE

John's drinking has become progressively worse over the years and his anger has seemed to escalate as well. He has made repeated attempts to stop drinking, but now no one in the family believes him when he begs forgiveness for his behavior and promises he will not drink again. The family members have adjusted their lives around the drinking. Sara, his wife, is always available to cover for him when needed and to conceal his tardiness or absences with excuses. She sometimes feels pride when she can resolve a seemingly impossible situation in a convincing manner. The children do not have friends come by on the weekends or holidays when their father particularly likes to drink. Everyone in the family "just knows" without it ever being spoken that no one is to tell their family health care provider about Dad's drinking. After all, John is a deacon at the local church and regarded highly in the community. You are surprised to read about John's arrest for driving under the influence. The next day, Sara comes to your office with severe depression, feeling that John's arrest is her fault.

Family issues that arise when a family member has an illness have some common characteristics. For example, in the family with a member who is an alcoholic, almost all family activities may be dependent upon the drinking behavior, or in the family with a member with chronic pain, all activity may be determined by the illness. Identity and development also can become entangled in the web of the problem and be constricted or stifled.

The family health care provider who understands the basic concepts of family dynamics understands how families attempt to adjust to challenges. For example, family boundaries may be closed as the family attempts to protect a member or conceal a problem.

Roles often shift, and communication patterns may break down. However, the resilience and strength of families to withstand enormous pressure and to incorporate stressors in a meaningful way is characteristic of many families. In addition, a crisis may move a family toward more intimacy and provide an opportunity for the positive growth of family relationships.

CHRONIC MEDICAL ILLNESS OR DISABILITY

Sally has spina bifida. Her parents have focused on her needs and have cared compassionately for her. Her sister, Jane, who is four years older, also is instructed by her parents to put Sally's needs first because "she does not have the opportunities and blessings you do." Often, Jane has to stay home and care for Sally or play with her instead of spending time with her own peers. Sally's mother continues to feel guilt that somehow she had not been as careful during her pregnancy with Sally as she should have been. She also wonders if God is punishing her through Sally's illness. Many of the activities of daily living that Sally could do for herself are done by her parents or Jane because they want to make life as easy as possible for Sally. The family also is reluctant to take advantage of respite care and other programs for families such as theirs. They plan on hiring a private teacher for Sally when she reaches school age. The family has maintained very closed boundaries since Sally's birth and accepts little support from others.

Sadly, Sally died at age thirteen. A year later, the parents divorced after a few months of very high conflict. You wonder how the situation might have been different if you had known the family earlier and had been able to encourage more expression of feelings, use of community resources, exposure to education about spina bifida, and balance in the family to address the needs of all members.

With the onset of an acute illness or sudden disability, families marshal their resources to meet the crisis. Often, this involves delaying certain activities until the family adjusts to the crisis. According to family stress theory, factors that mediate this adjustment include the availability of resources to meet the crisis, the extent of the crisis itself, and how the family interprets the problem and the meaning given to it. The family's past experiences dealing with crises or witnessing crises of friends and family can determine the trajectory of the response to acute illness or disability. A tightening of family boundaries often occurs or an opening for support from others as the family responds to an acute crisis.

The family's *explanatory model* or interpretive framework for understanding crises is important for the health care provider to understand. For example, if the family interprets the illness as punishment from God or understands disease as a weakness, the result could be blame and isolation of the sick person. Health care providers who focus only on the disease may miss the subjective experience and meaning of the illness for the individual and the family and thus miss the opportunity to be sensitive and supportive in a way that resonates with them.

Most families adjust when the acute phase is past or the disease is removed. However, even with acute illness or temporary disability, the family may become stuck in a more defensive mode and fail to regroup or return to a normal level of functioning. Health care providers need to assess how the family is adjusting or has adjusted to an illness or disability. Questions such as, "How has the illness or disability changed family life or activities?" "How do family members feel about the illness or disability?" or "What are the plans for dealing with the illness or disability?" can be important discussion points.

With an acute illness that becomes chronic or with permanent disability, the family is forced to make a long-term adjustment. According to the Centers for Disease Control, more than ninety million Americans live with chronic illness (CDC, available online at www.cdc.gov/ncdphp/overview.htm). Increasing longevity is predictive of an increase in chronic illness. Several questions can help health care providers understand how chronic illness is affecting the family.

1. How has the family reorganized itself or will it have to reorganize itself?
2. How have roles changed since the diagnosis?
3. Who has the primary responsibility for managing the disorder?
4. How do family expectations fit with those of the health care professionals?

5. Is the illness or disability openly discussed?
6. How has the family mood been affected by the illness? (Rolland, 1994, pp. 67, 72)

Many families must make significant adjustments to chronic illness. Grief, frustration, anger, and loss can be major components of such an adjustment. The roles of family members may also change. The individual who has been the primary wage earner may no longer be able to work, and another family member may become responsible for finances. Family rituals or recreational outings may no longer be feasible. Family life cycle events may be disrupted, or the family may have more difficulty moving through a life cycle stage. The following eight major issues for patients with chronic illness are also issues for their families:

1. control,
2. self-image,
3. dependency,
4. stigmatization,
5. abandonment,
6. anger,
7. isolation, and
8. death. (Pollin and Kanaan, 1995, pp. 47-98)

Chronic illness affects couple relationships by impacting relationship quality (e.g., chronic illness decreasing, increasing, and being unrelated to marital satisfaction), roles, and responsibilities, and social support (Kowal et al., 2003). Chronic illness affects the family as well. It can come upon any couple or family, however, improving relationships by interventions such as assisting with processing emotional experiences and comforting each other may act as a buffer from the onset of physical illness and the course of disease (Kowal et al., 2003).

When working with patients with chronic illness and their families, consider the following:

1. *Onset,* which can be acute (e.g., stroke, heart attack) or gradual (e.g., arthritis, Parkinson's disease)
2. *Course,* which can be progressive, constant, or relapsing

3. *Outcome,* which can be nonfatal or fatal
4. *Incapacitation,* which can be none, mild, moderate, or severe (Rolland, 1994, p. 23)

This typology can be used to prompt the health care provider to inquire about emotional responses to illness. In women, for example, activity limitations of disability may be indicative of potential depressive disorders (Chapman et al., 2001). This typology can assist with providing anticipatory guidance and encouraging the family to plan ahead.

Childhood chronic illness or disability results in greater risk for mental health problems in the child. Variables, such as child self-concept, intelligence, and life stress, can modulate or exacerbate adjustment (Cohen, 1999). Families with such children should be assessed for isolation, profound guilt, high levels of marital conflict, the effect of illness on siblings of the ill child, and stigmatization and discrimination by others (Benedetto and Olisky, 2001). Parents may feel ambivalent about their child—they may feel that they should not feel sad or angry about major changes in their child as a result of injury or disease because at least their child has survived (Logan and Sims, 2002).

As part of the normal adjustment to and acceptance of the illness or disability of a child, parents often question the diagnosis, treatment, and prognosis and may become frustrated with the complexity of the treatments or uncertainty of cure (American Academy of Pediatrics, 2001). Mutual, compassionate participation in decision making with the parents and answering questions regarding complementary and alternative treatments is essential. Often the aspects of the child's life that are still normal become obscured because of the illness or treatment. Therefore, assisting the parents to refocus on the normalcy in the child's life is essential (Benedetto and Olisky, 2001). Parents play a major role in determining how a disability will affect the family; assisting them in seeing the positive attributes of a child with a disability is essential (Olkin, 1999).

Early intervention services for children with disabilities and those at risk for disabilities are mandated by federal and state statutes (American Association of Pediatrics, 2001). Attending to each milestone of a child's life with anticipatory guidance and discussion can be a way to assist the family in meeting any difficulty with the transitions. For example, when a child with a disability starts school, the limitations may become more pronounced in the mind of the child or the parents.

The term *preinjury marriage* is used to describe a marriage that is in place before the occurrence of an injury or disability. *Postinjury marriage* describes a marriage that occurs after a partner's injury or disability. In either type of marriage, health professionals must not ignore the partner without the disability. When there is a disability in a couple's life, there is disequilibrium. Health care providers should consider how the disability changes family dynamics, such as roles, caregiving, and boundaries. When the individual with a disability gets married, his or her partner may have such qualities as independence, maturity, good communication skills, and may not be bound by society's stereotypes and stigmas regarding disability, thus providing better marital adjustment (Olkin, 1999).

Family support groups may be helpful. These help establish a community of families with shared experiences, emphasize family strengths and a nonpathologizing stance, allow for multiple perspectives on illness issues and management, and allow patients and their families an opportunity to observe other families from which new perspectives evolve (Steinglass, 1998).

DEMENTIA

By 2040, approximately 1 in 30 Americans, or approximately 9 million individuals, will have Alzheimer's disease, the most common form of dementia (Brody and Cohen, 1989). Other diseases, such as dementia associated with cerebrovascular disease, extrapyramidal features, and frontotemporal degenerations, cause another 20 to 40 percent of dementias (Knopman, 2001). Dementia influences many families.

The onset of dementia has been compared with the beginning of a new developmental stage for the family, and it is a critical transition point for family functioning (Mitrani and Czaja, 2000). The family health care provider who understands family dynamics will want to assess several areas of the family system interaction for adjustment and support mechanisms (see Exhibit 4.2). Additional family interactional patterns to note include the following:

1. Functions of leadership left void by the person with dementia (Is the family fulfilling these?)
2. Members who may usurp the caregiver (What power struggles are going on in the family?)
3. Communication in the family (Is the communication vague, overly intense, or lecture-oriented?)
4. Expectations of family members (Are the individual with dementia and the caregiver expected to function beyond their capacity?)
5. Degree of emotional involvement (What is the emotional overinvolvement or underinvolvement among family members?) (Mitrani and Czaja, 2000)

The stages of progression in dementia are defined as follows:

1. *Early stage*—Families must accept the diagnosis and its meaning and that no known cause and little hope of cure exist.
2. *Mid stage*—Families must cope with the individual's troubling and disrupting behaviors, such as confusion and wandering.
3. *End stage*—Families must provide terminal care. (Davis, 1997, p. 86)

Although the family may benefit from counseling at any time during the progression of the disease, it is especially helpful in the early stage when fears and reactions can be discussed. In addition, health care providers can provide anticipatory guidance and education that may prevent some misunderstandings and surprises at later stages of the disease. The family needs to decide legal matters early, while the affected individual can still make known his or her wishes with respect to a living will and guardianship.

Caregiver burnout is a risk associated with the care of family members with dementia. Even when respite care is available, it can be difficult for many caregivers to give themselves permission

EXHIBIT 4.2.
Assessing the Family Coping with Dementia

Family Education

- Have an initial family consultation, with key members of the family present.
- What do the family members know or need to know about the dementia at this time? Because of the stress of the care and the emotional factors involved, you may need to repeat information at various times.
- Anticipatory guidance for the future stages of the illness is imperative for proper plans and practical interventions (safety precautions, for example) of care to be accomplished.

Family Dynamics

- Do all members have a similar understanding of the stage of the illness? Misunderstandings can arise from family members who have less contact with the patient not realizing the extent or progression of impairment.
- Is a caretaker assuming all control of the patient's life instead of leaving the patient with as much autonomy and independence as is safely possible? Emphasize any normal abilities of the patient.
- How well does the family appear to work together with the same agenda?
- Are previous family conflicts and dynamics being exacerbated by the family stress?

Family Roles

- Who is the family manager of the care? Is the family consensus that this person be the manager? What emotional support from the family does this manager obtain?
- Who is the family "health expert"? This may or may not be a person medically trained, but maybe a person who can sabotage or support the physician's suggestions. As far as possible, the physician should attempt to have a positive relationship with the family "health expert" for the best of the patient.

- Is there a family agitator who is against everyone, including the physician? Rather than take this person on yourself, attempt to let the family deal with this person. Try to maintain a position that is not overly reactive to such a person.
- As is often the case in chronic care, it is important that the family should choose a spokesperson to facilitate interactions with health care issues.

Family Care

- The caregivers are the "hidden patients." Consider them a part of your care of the patient. Watch for signs of anxiety, depression, burnout, anger, and extreme overfunctioning.
- Check out emotions of caregivers such as shame, guilt, fear, frustration, and grief (loss of normal relationship with patient and then loss due to the patient's death).
- Watch for false hope and unrealistic expectations; do not remove these too quickly, but gradually educate.

Family Resources

- What outside resources are available in the community (community support organizations, religious institutions, respite care, extended family, friends, and financial)?
- Gradually educate and prepare the family to utilize Hospice as the terminal stage approaches.

to be away from the patient (Strang and Haughey, 1999). Health care providers may assist caregivers in giving themselves permission by helping to focus on how their caregiving ability will be enhanced if they replenish and renew themselves. In addition, health care providers can assist in discussing various options for caregiving, strategies for implementing these options, and potential problems of various arrangements (see Exhibit 4.2).

After the death of a person with dementia, the caregiver may feel ambivalent—relief followed by guilt about feeling relieved. Therefore, anticipating and discussing this with caregivers can be helpful. Caregivers often have a grief experience during the period of the loss of the person's cognitive abilities and again at the death of the family member (Almberg et al., 2000). Postdeath adjustment is influenced by the social support the caregiver has had while caring for the family member and during the bereavement period.

BEREAVEMENT

In recent decades, more deaths of terminally ill patients have occurred in hospitals than in homes, although this may be gradually reversing with the increased use of home-based health care. This has relieved families of some of the stressors of caregiving for family members who are dying, yet it also has been instrumental in making death seem unnatural.

Death can have profound effects on the surviving individuals, family systems, and communities. For the family, it may mean a disruption in the family life cycle and family balance. Some families, already stressed, may never return to good functioning. For example, the death of a child often precipitates the end of the parents' marriage (VanKaywyk, 1998). Other families may have a period of disorganization as they attempt to adjust to the death.

Another family loss that society often minimizes is the effect on parents and surviving siblings of a loss by a miscarriage. After a miscarriage, women frequently experience disturbing flashbacks, nightmares, suicidal ideation and suicide attempts, guilt, grief, and feelings of being overwhelmed and "going crazy" (DeFrain et al., 1996). Health care providers also should assess for sexual problems because fear of another pregnancy and miscarriage can create sexual dysfunction in these couples. One study found that the most immediate need from medical personnel when there was a pregnancy loss was to be encouraged to tell the pregnancy and loss story and be listened to and heard (Corbet-Owen and Kruger, 2001). One could surmise that intervening in this way with the couple or family, when possible, may lessen the potential of long-term complicated grieving.

Usually family members not only grieve as a family, but also grieve in individual ways and may not understand other family members who grieve differently. This can result in conflict and misunderstanding. For example, one family member may appear outwardly to be functioning as usual, while another is centered on the loss. Family members may be at different points in the grieving process.

Using available resources can be important to determining how a family responds to loss. Extended family support, financial resources, and community support can be vital during such times. Often, support is given initially until such time as others expect the family should be "getting over it." Withdrawal of support may then occur as these individuals go on with their own responsibilities of living. Spiritual beliefs may assist with the grief process: stronger spiritual beliefs appear to positively affect the course of bereavement (Walsh et al., 2002). Therefore, sensitively encouraging patients and their families to incorporate their religious faith into their grief experience or speak with their spiritual leaders may help provide a framework for how to better deal with their bereavement.

Some families have intergenerational patterns of grief and loss that may intensify current losses. These patterns may rigidify ways of reacting to loss or even day-to-day activities. For example, a family that has experienced the loss of a child in a prior generation may be overprotective and cautious with children of the current generation. Death can shift family triangles, coalitions, and alliances so that significant reorganization of the family system occurs even with a death in an older generation. Death often appears to give the impetus to a surviving family member to move toward marriage, new relationships, or pregnancy. Another way the legacy of past generational losses affects the current generation is the fear, conscious or unconscious, that an individual may have the same illness his or her parent had as he or she reaches the parallel age.

Assessing how a family deals with a terminally ill person is necessary. Often, there is *anticipatory grief* as the family members realize the ill member is dying. In some cases, the terminally ill begin to withdraw emotionally as death approaches, in an attempt to protect the family members. On the other hand, family members may begin to withdraw emotionally from the member who is dying as a self-protective measure without consciously being aware of what they are doing. This can leave the individual who is dying feeling even more isolated and alone.

Another form of bereavement, *traumatic grief,* has a cluster of symptoms of separation distress (e.g., yearning and excessive loneliness); traumatic distress (e.g., numbness); and loss of trust (Prigerson et al., 2001). Traumatic grief usually occurs after a partner who was in a close, supportive marriage has been widowed; this may put the survivor at risk for health problems. In addition, primary family members can experience intense distress when another family member dies a violent death. The family member may have traumatic responses, such as intrusive thoughts, flashbacks, and even dreams containing imaginary replays of the violent death (Rynearson and Favell, 2001). When a violent death occurs, screening family members for comorbid psychiatric disorders is essential.

The stage approach to grief derived from the work of Elisabeth Kübler-Ross (1969) is being challenged in the grief literature. One of the problems with the stage-based approach is that it tends to give the impression that there is a stepwise progression to grief when, in fact, grief can be manifested and expressed in many ways. Also, past models give the impression that grief resolves but, in fact, it often evolves but remains (Hagman, 2001). A poignant statement from a patient whose husband died three years prior sums up grief rather well: "The depth of my grief is not always with me, but the grief is never going to go" (Markowitz and Rabow, 2002, p. 882).

Facing the death of one of its members is one of the most intense struggles for a family. The pain, disruption, and disorganization can be tremendous. Health care providers can be a stabilizing influence for family members during such a crisis. Working with families in grief can be stressful, but it also can be one of the most rewarding aspects of the health care provider-patient relationship.

MENTAL ILLNESS

In addition to the challenges of dealing with a mentally ill individual, families with a member who is mentally ill must also deal with the stigma and misunderstandings associated with mental illness. Caring for chronically mentally ill family members can be gratifying, but caregivers who are men, lack family support, and who are younger, can experience significant distress and depression (Heru, 2000). Health care providers may not provide psychiatric treatment, but they do provide treatment for physical conditions and problems a mentally ill patient may require. Therefore, consideration of possible tensions in families with members who are mentally ill is of paramount importance.

Antagonistic *expressed emotion,* which is an attitude displaying high levels of criticism, hostility, and emotional overinvolvement toward the family member with a mental illness, is a predictor of relapse. Issues in families with a member with schizophrenia, and perhaps other psychiatric disorders, include the following:

1. Guilt about genetic transmission of the illness
2. Grief about losses for the family and individual due to the illness
3. Inadequacy about caring for the individual
4. Concern about dependency needs
5. Conflict among family members about how to deal with the family member with mental illness
6. Criticism or lack of acknowledgment by other family members about caregiving efforts
7. Feelings of helplessness and hopelessness (Bloch et al., 1995, pp. 416-418)

Providing education to families with a member who is mentally ill is important. Most want information about the mental disorder, symptoms, resources, respite care and services, and ways to reduce anxiety (see Resources).

ALCOHOLISM

Family dynamics have been incorporated into treatment of alcoholism for several decades. Family treatment has been validated as effective and family therapy can produce increased engagement and retention in treatment, reduced substance use, and enhanced marital and family functioning (Clark, 2003).

Health care providers recognize the reciprocal nature of how the family responds to a member who abuses a substance and how chronic use by a family member affects the family. A "dance," or interaction, occurs among members. An example of this is a cycle in which the alcoholic drinks and the nonalcoholic spouse responds with anger and criticism, then the alcoholic drinks more followed by the nonalcoholic spouse criticizing more. Roles and family life can begin to revolve around the substance abuse. The family dynamics can unintentionally reinforce or support the substance abuse problem and without attention to these dynamics interventions will likely fail (Clark, 2003).

Specific roles were observed in families in which a member abuses alcohol, such as the *enabler* (Wegscheider-Cruse, 1981). Enablers adjust to the substance abuse by becoming overly involved with the addicted person, such as in assisting and protecting the addicted person or, on the other hand, exhibiting open hostility while hindering any genuine forward movement (Liepman, 1994). Other family members may assume roles that attempt to make the family look good, such as a child who excels in school or athletics (the "family hero"), or dispel some of the tension in the family, such as the child who becomes known for making individuals laugh (the "family clown"). The danger in extremes of these roles is the resulting rigidity and denial of inner emotional needs.

Additional ways a family may be affected by the consequences of addiction are shifts in priorities, changes in values, illness and disability, violence, early death, lower levels of social support, and greater risk of transmission of the illness. A family history of alcohol and other drug abuse is one of the most powerful influences on a child's current and future health and well-being (Werner et al., 1999). Most primary care health care providers are familiar with the CAGE questionnaire as a substance abuse screening tool.

— C = Have you ever felt that you should cut down on your drinking?

— A = Have people annoyed you by criticizing your drinking?

— G = Have you ever felt bad or guilty about your drinking?

— E = Have you ever had a drink first thing in the morning to calm your nerves or to get rid of a hangover (**e**ye opener)? (Ewing, 1984, pp. 1905-1907)

A family-focused CAGE questionnaire, developed from the original CAGE questionnaire, broadens the questions to include all individuals in the family, not just the individual patient, and is more sensitive than asking about perceived family alcohol problems (Frank et al., 1992). The family-focused CAGE adds words that expand the CAGE to include family members in each of the CAGE questions so that the questions are not just asked about the person present.

—Have you ever felt that you or anyone else in your family should cut down on your/their drinking?
—Have you or anyone in your family ever felt annoyed by complaints about drinking?
—Have you or anyone else in your family ever felt bad or guilty about your/their drinking?
—Have you or anyone else in your family ever had a drink first thing in the morning to steady nerves or get rid of a hangover? (Frank et al., 1992, p. 212)

The scoring cut off is two or more positive answers for the family-focused CAGE screening instrument.

The family's reaction to treatment can be significant (McBride, 1988). When an alcoholic stops drinking, the family may have difficulty adjusting to his or her sobriety. The initial "honeymoon" stage where the family members are overjoyed that the family member has stopped drinking may be short-lived; this is especially true if the family members do not have education and guidance about the adjustments that sobriety may bring. One review of the literature mentioned how most families with alcoholic members would have serious "side effects" if permanent sobriety were achieved (Liepman et al., 1986). For example, the nonalcoholic spouse, who may have had to assume the role of being in charge and overinvolved, may have difficulty trusting and sharing authority in the family. Other family issues that had been ignored because of the focus on the alcoholism may now come to the fore-front with full force. Unfortunately, there is a high risk for divorce after sobriety.

Referral to Alcoholics Anonymous (AA) for the patient with a drinking problem, Al-Anon for the patient's family member or friends, and Alateen for the patient's children is important. These groups can help to normalize feelings, give support, and lessen the reactivity of family members. However, not all individuals will find that these organizations meet their needs. Encourage individuals attending such groups to try groups at various locations, if at all possible, because the group dynamics and personalities can vary considerably. Family therapy can be an important part of a treatment strategy and aid the family in recovery. In difficult cases, some professionals use an "intervention," where the person with the addiction is unexpectedly brought in and confronted by several significant individuals. However, not all individuals react to such confrontation in a positive manner, and professionals should only carry out such interventions if they have been trained for such or have the assistance of a counselor (see Resources).

HEALTHY FAMILIES

Becoming overly focused on finding pathology to the neglect of observing strengths and positive abilities in families is easy to do. However, many families manifest tremendous health and strength. Family strengths that may assist families through difficult transitions can be supported and encouraged. Six characteristics that have been identified in the research literature as qualities of strong families include the following:

1. Commitment, which involves the value and dedication given to each other
2. Appreciation and affection, which are expressed and felt often
3. Positive communication and good communication skills
4. Participation in family activities

5. Spiritual well-being, which gives meaning, purpose, and a sense of a greater good in life (this may or may not involve participation in a formal religion)
6. The ability to cope with stress and crises (Stinnett, 1999, p. 6)

Some families have a philosophy of life that assists them in navigating life's course in a positive manner. These families view life as a challenge, see crisis as opportunity, and believe that difficulties will eventually work out in a good way. Such families may bear great adversity and appear to adapt well (McBride, 1998).

The concept of resilience historically has been important in family therapy (Hawley, 2000). McCubbin and McCubbin use the concept of "family schema," which are the family's set of beliefs, to describe resilient families. Healthy family schemas emphasize such things as a collective "we" more than "I," show a willingness to accept less than perfect solutions to life's demands, and usually are confident about the ability to overcome difficult circumstances as a family (McCubbin and McCubbin, 1993).

The presidential report of the National Council on Family Relations (NCFR) titled "2001: Preparing Families for the Future" stated,

> American families today are diverse in terms of ethnicity, family dynamics, and type of family structure. The traditional family pattern—of husband, wife, and children in a nuclear family—has changed dramatically, and we see more single-parent families and stepfamilies across all cultural groups. Policies and programs must take family diversity into account, learn from it, and value the strengths it can provide. We must help families of all colors build on their unique strengths. (Olson and Hanson, 1990, p. 576)

This challenge also must be heeded by family health care providers.

A leading family therapist expressed the concept of the *intentional family*. The intentional family is defined as

> one whose members create a working plan for maintaining and building family ties, and then implement the plan as best they can. . . . At heart, the intentional family is a ritualizing

family. It creates patterns of connecting through everyday family rituals, seasonal celebrations, special occasions, and community involvement. (Doherty, 1999, p. 8)

Health care providers should capitalize on the resilience, strengths, and possibilities of families rather than focusing on family problems and dysfunction. At times, the health care provider is the key player in assisting a family to realize its own strengths and capabilities.

CONCLUSION

Understanding some of the system dynamics of families is necessary to assess and treat individual members. Boundaries, rules, roles, and communication dynamics in families tell us much about how they order and process their world. The family life cycle provides a way to organize thinking about families. Life cycle transitions are important because, at these critical movements, there is more potential for problems to occur. Health needs may vary across stages of the family life cycle.

Significant events (e.g., marriages, divorces, births, and losses) occur in family life and affect the family. Assessing how these events influence family members and how they are interpreted by the family can give the health care provider better tools for intervening and supporting the family during such times. Knowledge of special family issues (e.g., parenting, abuse, disability, and chronic illness experiences) gives the health care provider the ability to better understand family stressors.

The diversity of family lifestyles is greater today than at any time in this nation's history. Health care providers must be knowledgeable and sensitive to multiple ways of being a family. They must be able to deal with the issues presented by traditional, single-parent, multiracial, divorced, and same-gender families. The type of family structure alone does not automatically adversely affect well-being (Lansford et al., 2001).

Finally, the family's perceptions of ill health and beliefs associated with it are important avenues for better patient care. The family remains an essential context for understanding health care and behavior. Incorporating knowledge about family systems will assist the health care provider in working with much greater skill and ease.

Resources

The Family with Adolescents

English A. Reproductive health services for adolescents. Critical legal issues. *Osstet Gyneolo. Clin North Am.* 2000;27:195-211.

English A, Kenny KE. State Minor Consent Laws: A Summary. 2nd ed. Chapel Hill, NC: Center for Adolescent Health & The Law. 2003.

Weddle M, Kokotailo P. Adolescent substance abuse. Confidentiality and consent. *Pediatr Clin North Am.* 2002;49:301-315.

Gay and Lesbian Families

Healthy People 2010: Companion Document for Lesbian, Gay, Bisexual, and Transgender (LGBT) Health. San Francisco, CA: Gay and Lesbian Medical Association. 2001.

Adoptive Families

National Adoption Information Clearinghouse, 1250 Maryland Ave., SW, Washington, DC, 20024. Phone: (703) 352-3488 or (888) 251-0075. Available at http://www.naic.acf.hhs.gov/index.cfm.

Families Without Children

Childless by Choice, P.O. Box 695, Leavenworth, WA, 98826. Web site: http://www.northvalley.net/cbc/.

Intergenerational Families

Grandparents As Parents (GAP). This organization will help individuals network with other grandparents. Web site: http://www.ext.colostate.edu/pubs/consumer/10241.html. Phone: 213-595-3151.

Family Behavioral Issues in Health and Illness
Published by The Haworth Press, Inc., 2006. All rights reserved.
doi:10.1300/5621_05

Mental Illness

NAMI. National Alliance for the Mentally Ill, Colonial Place Three, 2107 Wilson Blvd., Suite 300, Arlington, VA, 22201-3042. NAMI Helpline: 1-800-950-NAMI (6264). Web site: www.nami.org/.

Alcoholism

Alcoholics Anonymous, Grand Central Station, P.O. Box 459, New York, NY, 10163. Web site: www.alcoholics-anonymous.org/.

National Association for Children of Alcoholics, 11426 Rockville Pike, Suite 100, Rockville, MD, 20852. Phone: 888-554-COAS (2627). Web site: http://www.nacoa.org.

Suggested Additional Important Reading

Becvar D, Becvar R. *Systems Theory and Family Therapy: A Primer.* 2nd ed. Lanham: University of America Press. 1999.

Carter B, McGoldrick M. (Eds.) *The Expanded Family Life Cycle: Individual, Family, and Social Perspectives.* 3rd ed. Boston: Allyn and Bacon, 1999.

Glick ID, Berman EM, Clarkin JF, Rait DS. *Marital and Family Therapy.* 4th ed. Washington, DC: American Psychiatric Press. 2000.

Gottman, M, Declaire D. *The Relationship Cure: A Five-Step Guide for Building Better Connections with Family, Friends, and Lovers.* New York: Crown Publishing, Inc. 2001.

Holloway RL (Guest Ed). *Behavioral Medicine in Family Practice. Clinics in Family Practice.* Philadelphia: W.B. Saunders Company. 2001;3.

McDaniel S, Campbell TL, Seaburn DB. *Family-Oriented Primary Care: A Manual for Medical Providers.* New York: Springer-Verlag. 1990.

References

Almberg BE, Grafstrom M, Winblad B. Caregivers of relatives with dementia: Experiences encompassing social support and bereavement. *Aging Ment Health.* 2000;4:82-89.

Amato PR. Life-span adjustment of children to their parent's divorce. *Future Child.* 1994;4:143-164.

American Academy of Family Physicians. Policy and Advocacy: Children's Health, 2002. Web site: http://www.aafp.org/x16320.xml. Accessed January, 2004.

American Academy of Pediatrics. Counseling families who choose complementary and alternative medicine for their child with chronic illness or disability. *Pediatrics.* 2001;107:598-601.

American Association of Pediatrics. Committee on Children with Disabilities. Role of the pediatrician in family-centered early intervention services. *Pediatrics.* 2001;107:1155-1157.

American Association of Pediatrics. Committee on Psychosocial Aspects of Child and Family Health. Coparent or second-parent adoption by same-sex parents. *Pediatrics.* 2002;109:339-340.

Anderson H. Feet planted firmly in midair: A spirituality for family living. In: Walsh F, ed. *Spiritual Resources for Family Therapy.* New York: The Guilford Press. 1999;157-176.

Baird MA. Introduction to family-oriented care in the new millennium. *Clin in Fam Prac* 2001;3:59-61.

Benedetto AE, Olisky T. Biracial youth: The role of the school counselor in racial identity development. *Professional Sch Counseling.* 2001;5:66-69.

Bloch S, Szmukler GI, Herrman H, Herman H, Benson A, and Colussa S. Counseling caregivers of relatives with schizophrenia: Themes, interventions, and caveats. *Fam Process.* 1995;34:413-425.

Bostock DJ, Auster S. Family Violence. Monograph, Edition No. 274. *Home Study Self-Assessment program.* Leawood, KS: American Academy of Family Physicians. 2002.

Brody J, Cohen D. Epidemiologic aspects of Alzheimer's disease: Facts and gaps. *J Aging Health.* 1989;1:139-149.

Family Behavioral Issues in Health and Illness
Published by The Haworth Press, Inc., 2006. All rights reserved.
doi:10.1300/5621_06

Bulick CM, Prescott CA, Kendler, KS. Features of childhood sexual abuse and the development of psychiatric and substance disorders. *British J of Psychiatry.* 2001;179:444-449.

Butler DJ, Lang F. When meeting with families. *Clin Fam Prac.* 2001;3:77-92.

Campbell TL. Family systems in family medicine. *Clin Fam Prac.* 2001; 3:13-33.

Carter B, McGoldrick M. Overview: The expanded family life cycle: Individual, family, and social perspectives. In: Carter B, McGoldrick M. (Eds.) *The Expanded Family Life Cycle: Individual, Family, and Social Perspectives,* 3rd ed. Boston: Allyn and Bacon, 1999;1-26.

Carter EA, McGoldrick M. (Eds.) *The Expanded Family Life Cycle: Individual, Family, and Social Perspectives.* 3rd ed. Boston, MA: Allyn and Bacon. 1999.

Centers for Disease Control and Prevention. Web site: http://www.cdc.gov/ncdphp/overview.htm. Accessed January, 2006.

Chapman DP, Campbell VA, Anda RF. Depressive disorders among women with disability. *Primary Care Psychiatry.* 2001;8:52-55.

Christie-Seely J. (Ed.) *Working with the Family in Primary Care: A Systems Approach to Health and Illness.* New York: Praeger. 1984.

Clark ME, Landers S, Linde R, Sperber J. The GLBT Health Access Project: A state-funded effort to improve access to care. *Am J Public Health.* 2001;91:895-896.

Clark W. Substance abuse and evidence-based family interventions. *Family Therapy Magazine.* 2003;2:15-19.

Cohen MR. Families coping with childhood chronic illness: A research review. *Fam Syst & Health.* 1999;17:149-164.

Cope J. Birth, childhood, adolescence. In: Wedding D, ed. *Behavior and Medicine.* 3rd ed. Seattle, WA: Hogrefe & Huber. 2001;135-160.

Corbet-Owen C, Kruger L. The health system and emotional care: Validating the many meanings of spontaneous pregnancy loss. *Fam, Syst & Health.* 2001;19:411-427.

Davis LL. Family conflicts around dementia home care. *Fam Syst & Health.* 1997;15:85-98.

DeFrain J, Millspaugh E, Xie X. The psychosocial effects of miscarriage: Implications for health professionals. *Fam Syst & Health.* 1996;14:331-347.

Doherty WJ. *The Intentional Family: Simple Rituals to Strengthen Family Ties.* New York: Avon Books. 1999;8.

Doherty WJ, Baird MA. *Family Therapy and Family Medicine: Toward the Primary Care of Families.* New York: Guilford. 1983.

Eggebeen DJ, Snyder AR. Children in single-father families in demographic perspective. *J Fam Issues.* 1996;17:441-465.

Ellis D. Safety, equity, and human agency: Contributions of divorce mediation. *Violence Against Women.* 2000;6:1012-1027.

Erikson E. *Childhood and Society.* New York: WW Norton & Company, Reissue edition. 1993.

Everett CA. (Ed.) *Family Therapy Glossary.* Washington, DC: American Association for Marriage and Family Therapists. 2000.

Ewing JE. Detecting alcoholism. The CAGE questionnaire. *JAMA.* 1984; 252:1905-1907.

Fields JM. America's Families and Living Arrangements. Current population reports, P-20; No. 537. US Bureau of the Census, Washington, DC. 2001:1-15. http://www.census.gov/prod/2001pubs/p20-537.pdf.

Foeman AK, Nance T. From miscegenation to multiculturalism. *J Black Stud.* 1999;29:540-558.

Frank SH, Graham AV, Zyzanski S, White S. Use of the Family CAGE in screening for alcohol problems in primary care. *Arch Fam Med.* 1992; 1:209-216.

Friedlander ML. Ethnic identity development of internationally adopted children and adolescents: Implications for family therapists. *J Marriage Fam Ther.* 1999;25:43-60.

Fuller-Thomson E, Minkeler M. African American grandparents raising grandchildren. *Health Soc Work.* 2000;25:109-118.

Gavagan T, Brodyaga L. Medical care for immigrants and refugees. *Am Fam Health Care Provider.* 1998;57:1061-1068.

Gay and Lesbian Medical Association. *Healthy People 2010: Companion Document for Lesbian, Gay, Bisexual, and Transgender (LGBT) Health.* San Francisco, CA. 2001.

Glick ID, Berman EM, Clarkin JF, Rait DS. Lesbian and gay couples. In: *Marital and Family Therapy.* 4th ed. Washington, DC: American Psychiatric Press. 2000;453-468.

Grilo CM, Masheb RM. Childhood psychological, physical, and sexual maltreatment in outpatients with binge eating disorder: Frequency and associations with gender, obesity, and eating-related psychopathology. *Obesity Research.* 2001;9:320-325.

Hagman G. Beyond decathexis: Toward a new psychoanalytic understanding and treatment of mourning. In: Neimeyer RA, ed. *Meaning Reconstruction & the Experience of Loss.* Washington, DC: American Psychological Association. 2001;13-31.

Hamberger LK. Spousal abuse in pregnancy. *Clin Fam Prac.* 2001;2:203-224.

Harrison AE. Primary care of lesbian and gay patients: Educating ourselves and our students. *Fam Med.* 1996;28:10-23.

Hawley DR. Clinical implications of family resilience. *Amer J Fam Ther.* 2000;28:101-117.

Heaton TB, Jacobson CK, Holland K. Persistence and change in decisions to remain childless. *J Marriage Fam.* 1999;61:531-539.

Hermon JH. Trauma and Recovery. *The Aftermath of Violence—From Domestic Abuse to Political Terror.* New York: Basic Books. 1992.

Heru AM. Family functioning, burden, and reward in the caregiving for chronic mental illness. *Fam Syst & Health.* 2000;18:91-103.

Hobbs F, Stoops N. Demographic Trends in the 20th Century. U.S. Census Bureau, Census 2000 Special Reports, Series CENSR-4, Washington, DC: U.S. Government Printing Office. 2002.

Ingersoll-Dayton B, Neal MB, Hammer LB. Aging parents helping adult children: The experience of the sandwiched generation. *Fam Relations.* 2001;50:262-271.

Janoff-Bulman R. *Shattered Assumptions: Towards a New Psychology of Trauma.* New York: The Free Press. 1992.

Johnson KO, Downs B. Current population reports: Maternity leave and employment of first-time mothers: 1961-2000. Washington, DC: U.S. Census Bureau. 2005;1-19.

Kahn NB Jr., corresponding author. Future of Family Medicine Project Leadership Committee. The future of family medicine: A collaborative project of the family medicine community. *Annals of Fam Med.* 2004;2, Supplement 1:S3-S32.

Kang DS, Kahler LR, Tesar CM. Cultural aspects of caring for refugees. *Am Fam Health Care Provider.* 1998;57:1245-1246, 1249-1250, 1253-1254.

Kelley SJ, Damato EG. When grandparents take on the parenting role. *Am J Nurs.* 1996;96:16.

Kirmayer LJ, Groleau D. Affective disorders in cultural context. *Psychiatr Clin North Am.* 2001;24:465-478.

Knopman DS. An overview of common non-Alzheimer dementias. *Clin Geriatr Med.* 2001;17:281-301.

Kowal J, Johnson SM, Lee A. Chronic illness in couples: A case for emotionally focused therapy. *J. Marital and Fam Therapy.* 2003;29:299-310.

Kramer L, Ramsburg D. Advice given to parents on welcoming a second child: A critical review. *Fam Relations.* 2002;51:2-14.

Kübler-Ross E. *On Death and Dying.* New York: Macmillan. 1969.

Lansford JE, Ceballo R, Abbey A, Stewart AJ. Does family structure matter? A comparison of adoptive, two-parent biological, single-mother, stepfather, and stepmother households. *J Marriage Fam Ther.* 2001; 63:840-851.

Lewis R, Yancey G, Bletzer SS. Racial and nonracial factors that influence spouse choice in black/white marriages. *J Black Stud.* 1997;28:60-78.

Liepman MR. The family with addiction. In: *Substance Abuse: Report of the Second Ross Roundtable on Critical Issues in Family Medicine in*

Collaboration with the Society of Teachers of Family Medicine. Columbus, OH: Ross Products Division, Abbott Laboratories. 1994;74-85.

Liepman M, White W, Nirenberg T. Children of alcoholic families. In: Lewis D and Williams C, eds. *Providing Care for Children of Alcoholics: Clinical and Research Perspectives.* Pompano Beach, FL: Health Communications. 1986;39-64.

Logan DE, Simms S. Relational approaches to crisis and conflicts in pediatric medical settings. *Fam Syst & Health.* 2002;20:61-73.

Markowitz AJ, Rabow MW. Caring for bereaved patients: "All the doctors just suddenly go." *JAMA.* 2002;287:882.

McBride JL. The Association Between Participation in Alcoholics Anonymous, Abstinence Patterns, Family Member Attendance of Al-Anon, Family Stress, and Family Functioning. Unpublished doctoral dissertation. The Florida State University. 1988.

McBride JL. Polarization could result in family medicine losing its (relational) soul: Reflections on Waters (2003) and commentaries by Armstrong and Holloway. *Fam Syst & Health.* 2004;22.

McBride JL. *Spiritual Crisis: Surviving Trauma to the Soul.* Binghamton, NY: The Haworth Press. 1998.

McBride JL, Armstrong G. The spiritual dynamics of chronic post traumatic stress disorder. *J Religion and Health.* 1995;34:5-16.

McCubbin MA, McCubbin HI. Family coping with health crises: the resiliency model of family stress, adjustment, and adaptation. In: Danielson C, Hamel-Bissell B, Winstead-Fry P, eds. *Families, Health and Illness.* New York: Mosby. 1993;21-64.

McDaniel S, Campbell TL, Seaburn DB. *Family-Oriented Primary Care: A Manual for Medical Providers.* New York: Springer-Verlag. 1990.

McGoldrick M, Carter B. Remarried families. In: Carter B, McGoldrick M eds. *The Expanded Family Life Cycle: Individual, Family, and Social Perspectives,* 3rd ed. Boston: Allyn and Bacon. 1999;417-435.

McGoldrick M, Gerson R, Shellenberger S. *Genograms: Assessment and Intervention.* 2nd ed. New York: WW Norton. 1999.

McQuillan J, Greil AL, White L, Jacob MC. Frustrated fertility: Infertility and psychological distress among women. *J Marriage and Fam.* 2003; 65:1007-1018.

Meurer JR, Meurer LN, Holloway RL. Clinical problems and counseling for single-parent families. *Am Fam Health Care Provider.* 1996;54:864, 867-870.

Miller BC, Fan X, Grotevant HD, Christensen MM, Coyl D, Van Dulmen MS. Adopted adolescents' overrepresentation in mental health counseling: Adoptees' problems or parents' lower threshold of referral? *J Am Acad Child Adolesc Psychiatry.* 2000;39:1504-1511.

Mills TL. Research on grandparent and grandchild relationships in the new millennium. *J Fam Issues.* 2001;22:403-406.

Mitrani VB, Czaja SJ. Family-based therapy for dementia caregivers: Clinical observations. *Aging Ment Health.* 2000;4:200-209.

Nichols W, Everett C. *Systemic Family Therapy: An Integrative Approach.* New York: The Guilford Press. 1986.

Nishimura NJ. Addressing the needs of biracial children: An issue for counselors in a multicultural school environment. *Sch Counselor.* 1995; 43:52-57.

Olkin R. *What Psychotherapists Should Know About Disability.* New York: Guilford Press. 1999.

Olson DH, DeFrain JD. *Marriage and the Family: Diversity and Strengths.* 3rd ed. Mountain View, CA: Mayfield. 2000.

Olson DH, Hanson MK. *2001: Preparing Families for the Future.* Minneapolis, MN: National Council on Family Relations. 1990.

Papadopoulos L, Bor R, Stanion P. Genograms in counselling practice: A review (Part 1). *Counseling Psychol Q.* 1997;10:17-29.

Parke RD. Beyond white and middle class: Cultural variations in families—assessments, processes, and policies. *J Fam Psychol.* 2000;14:331-333.

Perrin EC. Technical report: Coparent or second-parent adoption by same-sex parents. *Pediatrics.* 2002;109:341-344.

Pollin I, Kanaan SB. *Medical Crisis Counseling: Short-term Therapy for Long-term Illness.* New York: WW Norton. 1995.

Prigerson HG, Silverman GK, Jacobs SC, Maciejewski PK, Kasl SV, Rosenbeck RA. Traumatic grief, disability, and the underutilization of health services: A preliminary examination. *Primary Psychiatry.* 2001; 8:61-66.

Quarles CS, Brodie JH. Primary care of international adoptees. *Am Fam Health Care Provider.* 1998;58:2025-2032, 2039-2040.

Rolland JS. *Families, Illness, and Disability: An Integrative Treatment Model.* New York: Basic Books. 1994.

Rynearson EK, Favell JL. Bereavement after a violent death. *Primary Psychiatry.* 2001;8:70-72.

Shapiro AF, Gottman JM, Carrere S. The baby and the marriage: Identifying factors that buffer against decline in marital satisfaction after the first baby arrives. *J Fam Psychol.* 2000;14:59-70.

Sherry SN, Nickman SL. Adoption and foster family care. In: LeVine MD, Carey WB, Crocker AC, eds. *Developmental-Behavioral Pediatrics.* 3rd ed. Philadelphia, PA: Saunders. 1999;132-139.

Sinclair ND, *A Pastoral Response to Post-Traumatic Stress Disorder.* Binghamton, NY: The Haworth Press. 1993.

Slonim-Nevo V, Sharaga Y, Mirsky J. A culturally sensitive approach to therapy with immigrant families: The case of Jewish emigrants from the former Soviet Union. *Fam Process.* 1999;38:445-461.

Stein MB, Barrett-Connor E. Sexual assault and physical health: Findings from a population-based study of older adults. *Psychosomatic Med.* 2000;62:838-843.

Steinglass P. Multiple family discussion groups for patients with chronic medical illness. *Fam Syst & Health.* 1998;16:55-70.

Stinnett N. *Fantastic Families: 6 Proven Steps to Building a Strong Family.* West Monroe, LA: Howard Publishing. 1999;6.

Strang VR, Haughey M. Respite—A coping strategy for family caregivers. *West J Nurs Res.* 1999;21:450-471.

Thornton A, Young-DeMarco L. Four decades of trends in attitudes toward family issues in the United States: The 1960s through the 1990s. *J Marriage Fam Ther.* 2001;63:1009-1037.

VanKaywyk PL. Parental loss and marital grief: A pastoral and narrative perspective. *J Pastoral Care.* 1998;52:369-376.

Visher EP, Visher JS. *Therapy with Stepfamilies.* New York: Brunner/Mazel. 1996.

Walsh K, King M, Jones, L, Tookman A, Blizard R. Spiritual beliefs may affect outcome of bereavement: Prospective study. *BJM.* 2002;2:324,1551.

Wegscheider-Cruse S. *Another Chance: Hope and Health for the Alcoholic Family.* Palo Alto, CA: Science and Behavior Books. 1981.

Weihs K, Fisher L, Baird M. Families, health, and behavior. *Fam Syst & Health.* 2002;20:7-46.

Werner MJ, Joffe A, Graham AV. Screening, early identification, and office-based intervention with children and youth living in substance-abusing families. *Pediatrics.* 1999;103:1099-1112.

Whitehead BD, Popenoe D. The state of our unions 2005: The social health of marriage in America. New Brunswick, NJ: The National Marriage Project (Rutgers University). 2005. Web site: http://marriage.rutgers.edu/Publications/SOOU/SOOU2003.pdf. Accessed Janurary, 2006.

Whitman-Elia GF, Baxley EG. A primary care approach to the infertile couple. *J Am Board Fam Pract.* 2001;14:33-45.

Zubialde JP, Aspy JP. It is time to make a general systems paradigm reality in family and community medicine. *Fam Syst & Health.* 2001; 19:345-359.

Index

Page numbers followed by the letter "e" indicate exhibits; those followed by the letter "f" indicate figures.

Family Behavioral Issues in Health and Illness
Published by The Haworth Press, Inc., 2006. All rights reserved.
doi:10.1300/5621_07

Order a copy of this book with this form or online at:
http://www.haworthpress.com/store/product.asp?sku=5621

FAMILY BEHAVIORAL ISSUES IN HEALTH AND ILLNESS

_____ in hardbound at $29.95 (ISBN-13: 978-0-7890-2943-0; ISBN-10: 0-7890-2943-X)

_____ in softbound at $19.95 (ISBN-13: 978-0-7890-2944-7; ISBN-10: 0-7890-2944-8)

Or order online and use special offer code HEC25 in the shopping cart.

COST OF BOOKS_____

☐ **BILL ME LATER:** (Bill-me option is good on US/Canada/Mexico orders only; not good to jobbers, wholesalers, or subscription agencies.)

☐ Check here if billing address is different from shipping address and attach purchase order and billing address information.

POSTAGE & HANDLING_____
(US: $4.00 for first book & $1.50 for each additional book)
(Outside US: $5.00 for first book & $2.00 for each additional book)

Signature_____

SUBTOTAL_____

☐ **PAYMENT ENCLOSED: $**_____

IN CANADA: ADD 7% GST_____

☐ **PLEASE CHARGE TO MY CREDIT CARD.**

STATE TAX_____
(NJ, NY, OH, MN, CA, IL, IN, PA, & SD residents, add appropriate local sales tax)

☐ Visa ☐ MasterCard ☐ AmEx ☐ Discover
☐ Diner's Club ☐ Eurocard ☐ JCB

Account # _____

FINAL TOTAL_____
(If paying in Canadian funds, convert using the current exchange rate, UNESCO coupons welcome)

Exp. Date_____

Signature_____

Prices in US dollars and subject to change without notice.

NAME_____

INSTITUTION_____

ADDRESS_____

CITY_____

STATE/ZIP_____

COUNTRY_____ COUNTY (NY residents only)_____

TEL_____ FAX_____

E-MAIL_____

May we use your e-mail address for confirmations and other types of information? ☐ Yes ☐ No We appreciate receiving your e-mail address and fax number. Haworth would like to e-mail or fax special discount offers to you, as a preferred customer. **We will never share, rent, or exchange your e-mail address or fax number.** We regard such actions as an invasion of your privacy.

Order From Your Local Bookstore or Directly From
The Haworth Press, Inc.
10 Alice Street, Binghamton, New York 13904-1580 • USA
TELEPHONE: 1-800-HAWORTH (1-800-429-6784) / Outside US/Canada: (607) 722-5857
FAX: 1-800-895-0582 / Outside US/Canada: (607) 771-0012
E-mail to: orders@haworthpress.com

For orders outside US and Canada, you may wish to order through your local sales representative, distributor, or bookseller.
For information, see http://haworthpress.com/distributors
(Discounts are available for individual orders in US and Canada only, not booksellers/distributors.)

PLEASE PHOTOCOPY THIS FORM FOR YOUR PERSONAL USE.
http://www.HaworthPress.com   BOF06